WHY CALORIES COUNT

CALIFORNIA STUDIES IN FOOD AND CULTURE

Darra Goldstein, Editor

WHY CALORIES COUNT

From Science to Politics

Marion Nestle AND Malden Nesheim

UNIVERSITY OF CALIFORNIA PRESS

Berkeley   Los Angeles   London

University of California Press, one of the most distinguished
university presses in the United States, enriches lives around
the world by advancing scholarship in the humanities, social
sciences, and natural sciences. Its activities are supported by
the UC Press Foundation and by philanthropic contributions
from individuals and institutions. For more information, visit
www.ucpress.edu.

University of California Press
Berkeley and Los Angeles, California

University of California Press, Ltd.
London, England

Library of Congress Cataloging-in-Publication Data

Nestle, Marion.
Why calories count : from science to politics / Marion Nestle
and Malden Nesheim.
    p. ; cm. — (California studies in food and culture ; 33)
  Includes bibliographical references and index.
  ISBN 978-0-520-26288-1 (hardback : alk. paper)
    I. Nesheim, Malden C.   II. Series: California studies in
food and culture ; 33.
    [DNLM: 1. Energy Intake—physiology.   2. Diet.   3. Food
Industry.   4. Marketing.   5. Obesity—prevention & control.
6. Politics. QT 235]
613.2'3—dc23   2011044785

Manufactured in the United States of America

21   20   19   18   17   16   15   14   13   12
10   9   8   7   6   5   4   3   2

In keeping with a commitment to support environmentally
responsible and sustainable printing practices, UC Press has
printed this book on Rolland Enviro100, a 100% post-consumer
fiber paper that is FSC certified, deinked, processed chlorine-
free, and manufactured with renewable biogas energy. It is
acid-free and EcoLogo certified.

To the memory of Wilbur O. Atwater, 1844–1907

The publisher gratefully acknowledges the generous support of the Barbara S. Isgur Public Affairs Endowment Fund of the University of California Press Foundation.

CONTENTS

Introduction

When our then-editor at University of California Press, Stan Holwitz, suggested that we write a book about calories, we said yes right away. Consumption of too few or too many calories is an important—arguably the *most* important—cause of public health nutrition problems in the world today. Problems with calories affect billions of people in rich as well as poor countries. Consuming too few calories leads to malnutrition (undernutrition), which makes people more susceptible to infectious disease. The result is stunted growth, misery, and premature death in children and adults. More than a billion people, most of them in poor countries, go hungry for lack of food.

At the same time, just as many people in the world are consuming more calories than they need and becoming overweight and obese. The numbers of obese people are rising rapidly, even in the poorest countries. Obesity is now so common that the populations of some poor countries contain nearly equal numbers of people who are undernourished and overnourished. Obesity raises risks for any number of chronic diseases, most notably type 2 diabetes.

The health consequences of too many or too few calories threaten to overwhelm the resources of individuals, families, and health care systems. Countries can ill afford the costs of health care for obesity-related chronic or infectious diseases or to have large segments of their populations unable to work or function adequately. Some analysts even suggest that the health burdens of obesity alone may shorten overall life expectancy within the next few years.[1]

Despite widespread concerns about the health and economic consequences of obesity on the one hand and undernutrition on the other, correcting calorie imbalances presents social and economic challenges that few countries are prepared to meet. Calories, therefore, affect societies in ways that are political as well as personal.

Calories, of course, derive from food. But calories are a convenient way to say a great deal about food, nutrition, and health. For this reason, and because calories are so poorly understood, we thought it would be useful to research and write about calories in all of their dimensions—personal, scientific, and political. And because we are both consummate "foodies" who derive enormous pleasure from eating, we liked the idea of using calories as a way to think about these aspects of food.

Let's be clear from the beginning: this is not a diet book with a breakthrough scheme for losing weight and keeping it off. Instead, we try to provide an appreciation for what you are up against if you want to control your body weight in today's "toxic," obesity-promoting—or as we like to call it, "eat more"—food marketing environment.[2] We intend this book to give you the information you need to interpret food labels, diet claims, and your own reactions to this food environment. Knowledge, we argue, is not enough to counter the biological urge to eat or the subtleties of food marketing, but it is a powerful first step in developing weight-management strategies that work for your particular body, lifestyle, and food preferences.

We need to explain that both of us are or were professors in human nutrition departments, Marion Nestle at New York University and Malden Nesheim at Cornell. Our collaboration grew out of a previous project that culminated in a book about the pet food industry.[3] In working on that project, we discovered that we enjoyed researching and writing together and shared similar views of the strengths and limitations of nutrition science and its implications for dietary advice. In this book, the word *we* refers to the two of us and to our joint opinion.

THE FOOD CONTEXT

In considering this project, we were acutely aware that calories do not exist in isolation. They come from food. And along with calories, foods supply nutrients (vitamins, minerals, amino acids, essential fats), of which forty or more are required for life. To meet your body's needs for calories and nutrients, you do best when you vary, balance, and moderate your food intake. Eating a variety of foods balances the nutrients, meaning that you get enough of the ones you need. Foods contain a great many nutrients but in different proportions. If one food is low in a particular nutrient, others will compensate. If you typically vary the foods you eat, you really don't have to worry about nutrients. This leaves moderation as the central nutritional concern. Hence: calories.

One caveat: varying food intake takes care of nutrient needs only when the foods are of good nutritional quality. Processing removes nutrients from foods and often adds calories. Here we must introduce some terms nutritionists use to describe the nutritional quality of foods:

- *Nutrient density*: The proportion of nutrients in a food relative to its calories. Fruits, vegetables, whole grains, nuts, lean meats, and low-fat dairy products are nutrient-rich for their calories. Because fruits and vegetables often contain a great deal of water, which has no calories, they have an especially high nutrient density.

- *Calorie density*: The number of calories relative to the weight of a food. Fruits and vegetables provide few calories relative to their weight. Their calorie density is low.

- *Empty calories*: Calories accompanied by no or few nutrients. Sugar, alcohol, and highly processed "junk" foods are characterized by a low nutrient density as well as a high calorie density. Their calories are "empty."

"Real," "whole," or relatively unprocessed foods tend to be high in nutrients for their calories and low in calories for their weight. Diets based on such foods usually are adequate in essential nutrients and promote health. Nevertheless, the vast majority of health problems that result from inadequate or excessive food intake depend more on calories than on nutrients. We realize that what follows may sound like heresy coming from a couple of nutritionists, but unless diets are severely limited in variety or based largely on empty-calorie foods, nutrient intake is likely to be adequate when calories are adequate. This is especially true in today's era of nutrient fortification and nutritional supplements.

If you are eating too many calories, your diet is likely to be healthier if the calories come from real foods. But a healthful diet cannot fully protect you from the effects of overeating. When it comes to calories and body weight, how much you eat matters more than what you eat. Consider, for example, pre-Westernized Japanese and Mediterranean diets. The traditional rice-based diet in Japan was extremely high in carbohydrate and low in fat, while the traditional Mediterranean diet had a much higher proportion of fat (olive oil). People who ate those diets balanced their calories with physical activity. They did not eat more food than they needed, were highly active, and were rarely overweight. Although widely varying in composition, both diets promoted good health.

THE CONFUSION CONTEXT

That these points and much else about calories are not obvious constitutes a major rationale for writing this book. In our experience, people are so confused about calories that we have come to think of them as the C-word. Nobody wants to talk about them. They are poorly understood, and understandably so. You cannot see, taste, or smell them. The only way you can tell whether you are getting enough or too many is to observe their effects on your belt size or your weight on a scale. Most people have some vague idea that calories have something to do with putting on weight, but little intuitive grasp of the number in foods or what they do in the body. This, however, does not stop diet gurus, food advertisers, or government agencies from using the word all the time.

To pick our favorite example: In the 2004 film *Super Size Me!* (Marion's screen debut), a camera crew asks people at random on the street to define *calorie*. You watch respondents struggling to say something that makes sense. The film records some of the more amusing attempts, but its director, Morgan Spurlock, tells us that his crew could not find even one person who could come up with a reasonable definition.

Public confusion about calories is widespread, has been studied extensively, and is entirely understandable. Calories are tangible when measured in food or in the body, but such measurements can be done only in laboratories using equipment or techniques that are not available to the average person. The very definition of *calories* is nonintuitive. They are a measure of the energy in food and in the body, but "energy" is conceptually abstract. To get a feel for calories, you have to know how they are measured and what they do, neither of which comes up much in day-to-day life.

Even talking about calories is difficult. For starters, calorie counts are given in no less than *five* different units—calories, Calories, kilocalories, Joules, and kilojoules (along with their abbreviations, cal, Cal, kcal, J, and kJ). Which unit you use depends on whether you are a chemist, a nutritionist, or someone just looking at a food label and whether you live in the United States or someplace else. The bewildering terminology, which we sort out in chapter 1, is the result of history and geography, and not even scientists have an easy time with it.

THE MEASUREMENT CONTEXT

Calories in food are measurable, although not conveniently. Scientists also can measure calories used in the body, but even less conveniently. To do so, they must house study subjects in metabolic chambers, attach them to devices that measure oxygen use, or feed them specially labeled isotopes of water—all experimentally difficult and expensive. As we will discuss, other ways of determining calories in food or in the body are *estimates*. Some estimates are better than others, but they are inevitably imprecise.

In the United States, the estimates used to evaluate the number of calories in food were developed more than one hundred years ago by a Department of Agriculture scientist, Wilbur Atwater. Atwater Values—4 calories per gram for protein and carbohydrate, and 9 calories per gram for fat—still remain the basis of calorie counts on food labels. Throughout the last century and well into this one, investigators have attempted to improve the accuracy of these estimates. Despite their imprecision, Atwater Values remain in common use.

We think Atwater Values have survived to the present era because as calorie estimates they are good enough. Precise measurements are essential for research purposes but matter much less to daily eaters. If you cannot make laboratory measurements or enroll in a scientific study, you can only guess the number of calories you eat or use. Estimations work well enough for most purposes, and we will have much to say about how the difference between measurements and estimations applies to current theories of dieting and weight loss.

Because of the inability to make actual measurements of calorie intake and use, body weight is by far the best measure of calorie adequacy. Your body weight is the net result of the balance between the calories you eat and those you use, store, put out, burn off, or, more formally, "expend"—all terms we will use interchangeably—in metabolism and physical activity. Despite enormous day-to-day variation in calorie intake and output, people generally tend to remain at a relatively constant body weight. How this works is one of the great puzzles of calorie balance and one we address throughout this book.

How many calories should you be eating every day? This question also poses conceptual difficulties. You cannot tell from looking at a food how many calories it contains, because size does not indicate number. An apple, for example, can provide about the same number of calories as a teaspoon of salad oil. Apples are mostly water and have few calories for their weight—a low calorie density. Salad oil, in contrast, is concentrated fat. Only a few components of foods provide calories: proteins, fats, carbohydrates, and alcohol. Of these, fats provide the most. Food components such as vitamins, minerals, antioxidants, cholesterol, and water either do not provide calories or provide so few that their calories can be ignored.

It is next to impossible to guess the number of calories in meals in restaurants or at salad bars or dinner parties—unless you weigh the foods and know how they were prepared. How important imprecise estimates might be to weight maintenance is a question we also consider. Imprecision complicates not only personal dietary decisions but also government decisions about food policy. And imprecise estimates make public education about obesity an especially challenging task, particularly in light of today's "eat more" food environment.

THE ENVIRONMENT CONTEXT

Advice to maintain or to lose weight invariably includes two elements: eat less (translation: take in fewer calories) and move more (expend more calories). We like to add a third admonition: eat better (meaning eat this instead of that). Following this advice usually means replacing high-calorie foods with those lower in calories, or restricting one or another food component that achieves the same goal. But if you do not know how many calories you need or how many are in the food you eat, the meaning of "eat less" is uncertain. Indeed, when researchers ask people how many calories they habitually eat, most responders *underestimate* the number by an astonishingly large percentage—30 percent or more. People confronted with large food portions underestimate calories by even larger percentages. And most people overestimate their levels of physical activity, also by large percentages.

Overweight and obesity are serious public health concerns, not least because they are preventable. Much of this book is about the relationship of calories to body weight. If this relationship were simple, it would not take a book to deal with it. But as we continually emphasize, food and calories are more than physiological; they also have social, political, and economic dimensions.

In the United States, for example, rates of obesity began to rise sharply in the early 1980s. At that time, people must have begun to eat more, move less, or do both. How that happened involved changes in agricultural and economic policies that promoted greater food production. As we explain in chapter 21, more food meant that the number of calories available in the U.S. food supply rose from 3,200 per capita per day in 1980 to 3,900 twenty years later. With so much food available, food companies had to find new ways to sell products in a competitive marketplace. Food prices dropped, and people suddenly could afford to eat more food outside the home more often, in more places and in larger portions—all of which encouraged greater calorie intake. Eating more is good for business. Eating less is not.[4]

In seeking ways to maintain sales, food companies insistently promoted their products through the use of health and nutrient-content claims on package labels. Packages began to sport claims that their contents were free of fat, cholesterol, trans fat, salt, or sugar; contained vitamins or antioxidants; or were organic or could help prevent heart disease or immune disorders. Because people tend to interpret the meaning of such claims as "low calorie," health claims are calorie distracters.[5]

Calorie distracters lull people into forgetting how much they are eating. They convey the impression that what you eat matters more to body weight than how much you eat. Conveying this impression is the basis of the flourishing diet industry. Diet experts say that if you follow their particular newly discovered dietary principle, often based on complicated metabolic reasoning, you will lose weight without having to give a thought to calories or how much you eat. Remarkably, the particulars of breakthrough diet plans vary and contradict one another. Some emphasize avoiding fat, while others say you should avoid carbohydrate. Still others focus on fiber or a particular food group. To the extent that these plans help you take in fewer calories, they will result in weight loss—at least as long as you stick to the plan, a challenge in itself.

We need to reemphasize that calories occur within the context of food, diet, culture, and lifestyle. The effects of calories must be understood within this broader context. Much evidence demonstrates the health benefits of consuming diets based on foods of high nutrient and low calorie density. Such diets are well established to meet nutrient needs as well as to reduce risks for heart disease, cancers, and other chronic diseases. They also make it much easier to balance calories and prevent weight gain.

ABOUT THIS BOOK

What we attempt to do here is to give you information you can use to interpret current concerns about calories as they relate to the full spectrum of calorie intake—from too little to too much—and the consequences of such concerns for food and nutrition policy. Much of the current debate about calories centers on just a few questions:

+ Why do some people and not others get fat, even though they eat similar diets?
+ How much do you have to overeat or undereat to gain or lose weight?
+ Why is it so much easier to gain weight than to lose it?
+ Which is more important to body weight and health, calorie intake or the composition of the diet?
+ Who is more responsible for childhood obesity: parents or society?
+ What is the role of government in ensuring that people have enough to eat?
+ What is the role of government in regulating the food environment and promoting appropriate calorie intake and expenditure?

Our approach to dealing with these questions begins with the science—how it developed, how it is used, and where it now stands. Because science necessarily occurs within the context of society, these questions also have evident social and political implications. We address these implications throughout this book.

Our purpose here is to give you a greater appreciation of calories and, as a result, of the pleasures and health-giving qualities of food. We hope that by understanding calories you will worry about them less, eat more healthfully without having to think about it, and enjoy your food even more. We also hope to inspire you to appreciate the political dimensions of calories and to press for policies that will make it easier for you and everyone else to have enough to eat, to eat better, and to be more active.

PART ONE

Understanding Calories
It All Starts with the Science

In thinking about how to begin a book about calories, we kept coming back to the science. Both of us were trained as scientists, Malden in nutrition and biochemistry and Marion in molecular biology and public health nutrition, and we tend to think like scientists. By this we mean that we consider as much of the available evidence as we can as a basis for forming opinions about diets and dieting. Doing this is not as simple as it might appear. Nutrition is an unusually challenging field of scientific inquiry. Human diets and behavior are difficult to investigate. People vary. Diets vary. Activity levels vary. The effects of what you eat now might not show up for decades. Your health and longevity depend not only on genetics but also on how your particular genetic makeup interacts with everything you eat, drink, and do, as well as with the social, cultural, physical, and economic environment in which you live.

Accounting for such variables requires putting people in controlled—virtually imprisoning—environments for as long as they can stand it. Nobody enjoys being treated like an animal in a cage, and few people are willing to subject themselves to controlled diets or environments for very long. Well-controlled dietary trials are expensive and tedious to conduct, monitor, and evaluate and generally can include only small numbers of study subjects. For practical reasons, most nutrition studies depend on analyses of self-reported accounts of dietary intake and physical activity. To say that such accounts are unreliable is to seriously understate the situation.

Consequently, studies of human nutrition require careful interpretation. Interpretation requires interpreters. Interpreters are humans too and bring their own experience, prejudices, and biases into the way they view study results. We do too. The fiercest arguments about calories—does what you eat matter more than how much you eat, and do small differences in estimates of the calories in foods make any difference to body weight?—depend on how the science is interpreted. Throughout this book, we present the science as we see it and provide references to our sources in the notes so you can read them and form your own opinion.

Scientific information is often abstract and technical, but we think the science of calories should be understandable to anyone willing to give it a try. To make the technical material easier to follow, we have divided the book into short chapters, each designed to address a question you might have about calories. We define new terms as we go along, and we keep abbreviations to a minimum.

In this first part of the book, we explain what calories are, relate the history of how they came to be understood, and describe how they are measured. We present this material first because everything in the rest of the book depends on it. If you are not trained in science, some of this material may be new to you. We encourage you to persevere. Whatever effort you put into understanding the science now will pay off later as you read our chapters on diets, dieting, and the politics of calories. Welcome to *Why Calories Count: From Science to Politics.*

CHAPTER 1

What Is a Calorie?

In embarking on an entire book about calories, we have to begin at the beginning—what to call them. Calories are units of work or heat, but what they are called depends on who is doing the calling. We think the name inconsistencies can be so confusing that we summarize them in table 1. We believe there is an easier, commonsense way to think about the definition, as we will explain. To get to that point, let's begin with the official definition used by chemists:

> One calorie is the amount of heat energy needed to raise the temperature of one gram of water by one degree centigrade, from 14.5° to 15.5°, at one unit of atmospheric pressure.

As a first step toward arriving at a more intuitive definition, let's ignore the ambient temperature and atmospheric pressure, as they usually do not make much difference except to scientists. But pay close attention to the weight units. In table 1, we emphasize *gram* in this definition to distinguish it from definitions based on heating an amount of water 1,000 times greater—a kilogram. A gram is about one quarter of a teaspoon. A kilogram is 2.2 pounds.

Gram units are inconvenient for most Americans, and so are so-called small calories, based on a gram standard. If food labels listed calories by the chemists' definition, your daily calorie requirements might be about 2,500,000 a day rather than 2,500, and a carrot would provide 25,000 calories instead of 25. That is why nutritionists much prefer to use kilocalories (kcal),

TABLE I TERMS USED TO REFER TO THE ENERGY VALUE OF FOOD

Used by	Term	Definition	Metric system equivalent
Chemists	calorie (cal), also called gram-calorie, g-calorie, or small calorie	Heat energy needed to raise the temperature of 1 gram of water by 1 degree C, from 14.5° to 15.5°, at 1 unit of atmospheric pressure	4.2 joules (J)
Physiologists, other scientists	kilocalorie (kcal), also called kilogram-calorie, kg-calorie, or large calorie	Heat energy needed to raise the temperature of 1 kilogram of water by 1 degree C, from 14.5° to 15.5°, at 1 unit of atmospheric pressure (identical to Calorie)	4.2 kilojoules (kJ)
U.S. nutritionists, federal regulators	Calorie (Cal), also called large calorie*	Heat energy needed to raise the temperature of 1 kilogram of water by 1 degree C, from 14.5° to 15.5°, at 1 unit of atmospheric pressure (identical to kilocalorie)	4.2 kilojoules (kJ)
International (metric) System of Units	joule (J)	A unit of energy equal to the work done by a force of 1 newton acting through a distance of 1 meter.[†]	0.24 cal
International system	kilojoule (kJ)	1,000 joules	0.24 kcal or Cal
International system	megajoule (MJ)	1,000 kilojoules	240 kcal or Cal

NOTE: Figures are rounded off from 4.184 J or kJ, and 0.239 cal, kcal, or Cal. A kilogram is 2.2 pounds.

*This is the term used on food package labels.

[†] For the record, 1 newton is equal to the force that would give a mass of 1 kilogram an acceleration of 1 meter per second per second.

units that are 1,000 times larger and based on the heat required to raise the temperature of a kilogram of water by one degree centigrade.

Here is where things get tricky. Because it feels awkward to say *kilocalories*, nutritionists shorten it to *Calories*, spelled with a capital C. Food labels list Calories, but they really mean kilocalories (also known as large calories or kilogram-calories). When spoken, *Calories* (capital C) and *calories* (small c) sound the same. As a result, when discussing the energy value of food, the words *kilocalories* (kcal), *Calories* (Cal), and *calories* (cal) have come to mean exactly the same thing: 1,000 chemists' calories. Hence: confusion.

The peculiar result of all this is that the word *calories* can mean two things at the same time: chemists' calories and nutritionists' Calories, which are 1,000 times greater. In common practice, most people use *calories*, capitalized or not, to mean kilocalories or Calories, despite the confusion this causes.

James Hargrove, who has written a fine history of the evolution of the terms, argues that "it is untenable to continue to use the same word for different thermal units (gram-calorie and kilogram-calorie) and to use different words for the same unit (Calorie and kilocalorie). The only valid use of the Calorie is in common speech and public nutrition education."[1]

We, as it happens, are in the business of public nutrition education, and we use common speech all the time. We do not view this situation as untenable, just confusing. The various definitions lead to problems that can be amusing or annoying, depending on how you look at them. For example, Hargrove points to the inconsistent use of the terms *calories* and *kilocalories*—in this case meaning the same thing—in the U.S. Code of Federal Regulations rules for food labels: "A normal serving of the food contains at least 40 kilocalories (that is, 2 percent of a daily intake of 2,000 kilocalories). . . . The food contains all of the following nutrients per 100 calories based on 2,000 calorie total intake as a daily standard."[2]

Public nutrition educators that we are, we follow common speech. Throughout this book we use *calories*, spelled with a small c, to refer to kilocalories/ Calories, unless we have a specific reason to use a more precise term. Food labels do this too.

JOULE CONFUSION

With this said, we must now introduce another source of confusion. We live in the United States. Practically everywhere else in the world, people use the metric system and follow the metric-based International System of Units (Système International d'Unités). In this system, food energy is expressed in joules or in their thousandfold-larger counterpart, kilojoules. We give the conversion factors in table 1. These terms also are used imprecisely, and we hear people talking about joules when they really mean kilojoules.

The easiest way to think of the conversions is to remember that 100 calories is about 420 kilojoules (or calories times 4.2) and that 2,400 calories is equivalent to 10,000 kilojoules. If you only want estimates, you can multiply calories by 4 to get kilojoules or divide kilojoules by 4 to get calories. This is obviously imprecise but should work well enough for most purposes. As you will soon see, "works well enough for most purposes" is a constant theme in this book.

And just for the record, let's add one more term. Nutrition scientists like to use *megajoule* (MJ) to describe energy intake or expenditure because it doesn't require as large a number. A megajoule is 1,000 kilojoules. A diet of 2,400 calories a day has 10,000 kJ or 10 MJ.

When the U.S. Food and Drug Administration wrote regulations for Nutrition Facts labels on food products in 1993, it seriously considered including both kilojoules and calories in the design but eventually rejected the idea, reasoning that no attempt to induce Americans to use the metric system has ever succeeded.[3] The historian Hargrove is thoroughly fed up with all this. He recommends getting rid of everything having to do with calories and switching to joules instead. Good luck with that. We doubt this will happen within our lifetime or even that of our children. In the meantime, we think *calories* works pretty well, once you get a feel for what they are. To that end, we invite you to take a look at our approach to understanding them more intuitively.

GETTING A FEEL FOR CALORIES

Our first recommendation is to convert the chemists' definition of Calories/kilocalories to something more convenient. We have already gotten rid of temperature and pressure. Let's now convert metric units to common household measures. A liter of water weighs about one kilogram and is almost the same volume as a quart (one liter equals 1.06 quarts). We think it is fair to say:

A calorie is about the amount of heat needed to raise the temperature of a quart of water by 1°C.

One food calorie isn't very much in diets of 2,000 to 3,000 a day. It makes more sense to deal with 100 calories. This is the amount in 100-calorie packs of snack foods, obviously, but also in a pat of butter, an apple, an 8-ounce soft drink, or two Oreo cookies. If 1 calorie raises the temperature of a quart of water by 1°C, then:

100 calories raises the temperature of one quart of water by 100°C.

One more tweak and we'll be done: 100°C is the same as 212°F—the boiling point of water. Here, at last, is our easy definition.

100 calories is the amount of heat needed to bring a quart of water to the boiling point.

What? You may feel warm after eating a big meal, but not *that* warm. Bodies contain about six quarts of blood. Why doesn't your blood boil when you devour a 600-calorie cheeseburger? The answer: metabolism. Metabolism, as we explain in chapter 5, taps off that heat in tiny increments to maintain body temperature and to power the digestion of food, the construction of new body molecules, and the action of muscles. Any energy you don't need right away gets stored, mostly as fat, to be used later, when you aren't eating.

HEAT CONFUSION

Basic ideas about how calories work in food and in the body are quite straightforward, if somewhat abstract:

+ Calories are units of energy.
+ Energy is the capacity to do work.
+ Work can be chemical (biochemical, in this case) as well as physical (muscular).
+ Biochemical reactions and muscle activity produce heat.
+ Heat can be measured as calories.

Food provides energy that fuels the work that bodies do: breathe, circulate blood, keep warm, transmit nerve impulses, excrete waste, move. Scientists measure the overall energy required for this work by the heat it produces, which they report in units of calories. This is much the same as the use of temperature to indicate the heat of the surrounding air. You know intuitively that you are going to shiver when the outside temperature is 20 degrees Fahrenheit but will be sweating if it is 100 degrees. Similarly, you can intuit that 100 calories doesn't represent very much food energy, whereas 5,000 is more than you are likely to need in a day.

If the notion of calories as a measure of heat does not seem obvious, it is surely because you cannot have a physical sense of them in food. Calories, recall, have no smell, taste, or appearance. Invisible as they are, you can only measure them with complicated equipment or tests or deduce them from what they do to your body weight.

The calories in a food are measured through the heat it produces when burned. This leads to one other potential source of confusion—the difference between energy, heat, and calories. Energy, defined as the capacity to do work, exists in different forms: heat energy, electrical energy, chemical energy, mechanical energy. In physics, the first law of thermodynamics states that these various forms of energy are completely interchangeable. Any form of energy can be converted into any other form. The steam engine is the obvious example: it uses the heat generated by burning fuel to produce steam that creates mechanical work.

Bodies also interconvert forms of energy. The chemical structures of certain food molecules—proteins, fats, and carbohydrates (and alcohol, which we will get to in chapter 11)—store energy. Metabolism transforms some of the chemical energy stored in food components into heat energy through a series of biochemical reactions that involve the oxygen you breathe. These are called *oxidation* reactions. We will say more about them in chapter 5. Metabolism also transforms food energy into mechanical energy in muscles and into electrical energy in the brain and nervous system.

Heat energy may appear confusing because you can measure it in two ways. You can stick a thermometer into a roasting turkey or a feverish child to measure internal heat. But to measure the energy stored in foods or expended in physical activity, you must use special devices or chemical techniques (see chapters 3 and 4). To summarize:

+ *Energy* is the capacity to do work. Food stores energy in the chemical structures of some of its molecules, mainly proteins, fats, and carbohydrates but also alcohol.

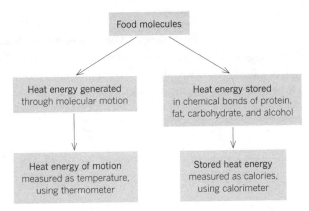

FIGURE 1. Food molecules produce heat energy in two ways: through molecular motion (measured as degrees Fahrenheit or centigrade) and through storage in chemical bonds (measured as calories).

- *Heat* is one form of energy, and the one most easily measured using a thermometer or devices that permit calories to be calculated.

- *Temperature* is a measure of the heat energy produced by the internal atomic motion of molecules of air, water, or other matter, as indicated on centigrade (Celsius) or Fahrenheit thermometer scales.

- *Calories* and *joules* are units of heat or work energy measured in experiments using calorimeter devices or through calculations based on chemical techniques.

Because heat is common to all of these measurements, we thought the diagram in figure 1 might help clarify the distinctions.

The diagram distinguishes energy produced by the motion of *all* molecules of food from the energy stored in the chemical bonds of the *particular* molecules that yield calories. The atoms in all molecules move to some extent, and the heat generated by that movement can be transferred to other molecules. Thermometers measure that transferable heat.

But only some molecules—proteins, fats, carbohydrates, and alcohol—store energy that can be metabolized and used to support life. The energy of motion and the energy stored in chemical bonds are different. Here is one way to think of the distinction: from the standpoint of metabolism and body weight, french-fried potatoes served steaming hot right out of the fryer have the same number of calories stored in their proteins, fats, and carbohydrates as they do when refrigerated or frozen.

In speaking about the energy content of foods and the effects of food energy in the body, we try to be consistent about using *heat* as one form of energy and *calories* as a way to measure the amount of heat energy. With the main sources of calorie-related confusion exposed, if not resolved, we can now take a brief look at how scientists came to understand all this.

CHAPTER 2

The History

From Ancient Greece to Modern Calorie Science

Although it may seem self-evident that food is essential to life, scientists did not have much real understanding about how food energy keeps bodies warm, growing, and functioning until the late 1700s. The earliest understanding of calories as energy released by the interaction of oxygen with food molecules is usually attributed to Antoine Lavoisier, who lived and died in the eighteenth century. Lavoisier's view of metabolism as an oxidation process—the "burning" of food molecules in the presence of oxygen—still holds true.

We explain how this works in later chapters, but to jump-start the discussion let's begin with a quick overview of the basic concepts. The three energy-producing molecules in foods—proteins, fats, and carbohydrates—are highly structured. Creating them takes energy, some of which gets stored in their chemical bonds. Once eaten, food molecules are attacked by digestive enzymes. Enzymes break the organized structures into pieces small enough to be absorbed through the wall of the digestive tract. As we illustrate in chapter 5, enzymes disassemble complex molecules of starch, for example, into simple sugars, a process that releases small amounts of energy.

During metabolism, enzymes further disassemble the absorbed sugars into even smaller pieces, releasing more energy. Other enzymes transfer some of this energy to small storage molecules. When the body needs energy, still other enzymes split the storage molecules to release it. The released energy powers the chemical reactions that create new body molecules or make muscles contract, and some of it keeps the body warm.

The chemical reactions involved in these processes are "oxidation" reactions. They require oxygen, which is obtained through respiration. You breathe in oxygen. You exhale carbon dioxide as waste. Your other metabolic waste product is water, which you mostly excrete in urine. Food molecules that are completely "burned" in the body end up as carbon dioxide and water. All of these processes yield heat.

Scientists now know a great deal about the chemical structure of food and each of the processes crucial to obtaining energy from food: digestion, absorption, metabolism, respiration, and excretion. We'll examine them all in subsequent chapters. But first, it's worth exploring why it took such a long time to figure out the role of food in the body.

ANCIENT IDEAS ABOUT FOOD ENERGY: HIPPOCRATES AND GALEN

The most important early writings about energy and body heat are attributed to the Greek physician Hippocrates (~460–370 B.C.).[1] Because the authorship of ancient texts is uncertain, the writings of Hippocrates are generally considered to include not only those of the physician himself but also those of his contemporaries and followers. In that sense, *Hippocrates* is something of a collective term. The writings, however, come across as if written by a single person, one who tried hard to make sense of his observations but sometimes jumped to conclusions that do not always make sense in modern terms. Even when his observations are right on target, he can sound much like a present-day diet guru.

Here, for example, he boasts of having been the first to discover the secret of health—balancing diet and activity: "This discovery reflects glory on myself its discoverer, and is useful to those who have learnt it, but no one of my predecessors has even attempted to understand it though I judge it to be of great value in respect of everything else. It comprises prognosis before illness and diagnosis of what is the matter with the body, whether food overpowers exercise, whether exercise overpowers food, or whether the two are duly proportioned. For it is from the overpowering of one or the other that diseases arise, while from their being evenly balanced comes good health."[2]

Hippocrates produced aphorisms, among them "Growing creatures have most innate heat, and it is for this reason that they need most food, deprived of which their body pines away." This particular statement was singled out by the twentieth-century nutrition scientist Graham Lusk as the earliest understanding of the role of calories in the body. Hippocrates also recognized that dietary prescriptions had to be tailored to individuals: "The various ages have different needs. Moreover, there are the situations of districts, the shiftings of the winds, the changes of the seasons, and the constitution of the year."[3] Whether such pronouncements made sense or not, they stayed in print, repeatedly translated—and famously mistranslated—from Greek into Arabic and Latin, and back again into Greek.

Five centuries later, Galen (~130–200), a Roman physician of Greek origin, translated the Hippocrates texts himself and became a devoted disciple. In prolific writings, Galen paraphrased (or plagiarized, if you prefer) Hippocrates, adding his own commentaries. He repeated much of what Hippocrates said about the digestion of common foods, their speed of passage through the body, and—apparently an issue of great concern—their propensity to produce flatulence. Hippocrates found turnips, for example, to be "heating, moistening, and disturbing to the body" but unable to "pass easily, either by stool or by urine." Galen solved this problem by insisting that turnips be cooked; otherwise, a turnip is "difficult to concoct [digest], flatulent, and causes loss of appetite, and sometimes gnawing sensations in the stomach." Despite what we would now consider minor—and sometimes major—errors in fact and interpretation, Galen sharply criticized anyone who disagreed with his or Hippocrates's views: "My opinion—and I swear to it by God—is that Hippocrates has made this account of his so clear and obvious that not even a child, much less anyone else, should find it obscure."[4]

The vehemence of these opinions would be of interest only to classical scholars except for one distressing historical fact. The writings of Hippocrates and Galen, no matter what they said, were accepted as indisputable by subsequent generations. Their ideas so dominated medical practice from the fifth century B.C. until the eighteenth century A.D. that science could make little headway. Hippocrates and Galen, for example, favored bloodletting as a treatment for many diseases. Although this practice is certain to increase calorie needs—if not cause anemia, infections, or death—it continued as *routine* medical treatment until well into the nineteenth century.

ORIGINS OF CALORIE SCIENCE

Fast-forward through the Middle Ages and Renaissance to the Enlightenment and the onset of the modern scientific era. To grasp how food provides energy and how the body uses it, scientists had a great deal of work to do. They first had to discover:

+ oxygen and carbon dioxide
+ the role of these gases in respiration
+ the relationship of food components to heat
+ the chemical conversions involved in digestion and metabolism
+ the chemical composition of foods

These discoveries were gradually accomplished and accumulated during the seventeenth to twentieth centuries. We summarize this lengthy history in appendix 1.

Santorio Sanctorius of Padua gets credit for the first fumblings toward a scientific understanding of human energetics—the use of energy in and by the body. In the 1600s, perhaps suffering from some kind of obsessive-compulsive disorder, he weighed himself, everything he ate and drank, and everything he produced in urine and feces nearly every day for thirty years. From these observations and measurements, Sanctorius observed the effects on his body of the difference in weight between the foods he ate and the waste products he excreted. He attributed this difference to "insensible perspiration." Figure 2 illustrates the weighing chair he designed for this purpose.[5]

True modern understanding of human energetics begins with the revolution in scientific thinking that accompanied the political revolution in France in the late 1700s.[6] Antoine Lavoisier, a French aristocrat, was its best-known scientific revolutionary. He constructed a device large enough to permit measurements of the heat produced by a living animal, in this case, a guinea pig. From experiments using such "whole-body" calorimeters, he concluded that animal respiration is a form of oxidative combustion, just like the burning of a candle. Both, he said, require oxygen. Both release carbon dioxide and water.[7] These promising investigations ended prematurely. Lavoisier was arrested during the deadliest days of the French Revolution and guillotined.

At about the same time in England, Adair Crawford was performing similar investigations with similar results. Although neither Lavoisier nor Crawford used the word *calorie* to describe animal heat, Lavoisier came close. He called his measurement device a calorimeter (*calorimètre*) and used terms such as *calorique* (caloric) and *chaleur* (heat) to describe his observations of animal metabolism. The first record of the use of *calorie* in its present sense as

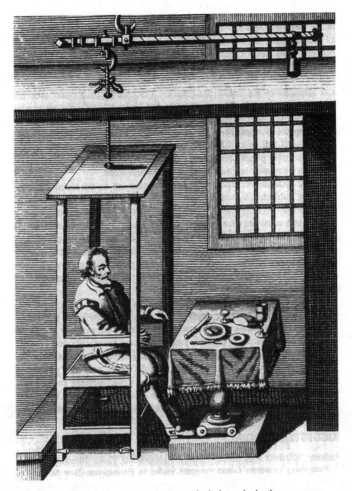

FIGURE 2. Santorio Sanctorius sitting in the balance he built to measure the effects of his food intake on body weight. Source: Quincy, 1718 (see note 5). Wellcome Library, London, used with permission.

a measurement of body heat dates to notes taken from lectures by the French scientist Nicolas Clément in 1824. Max Rubner in Germany gets credit as the first scientist to publish the use of the term in its modern sense.[8]

German physiologists of the mid-1800s, such as Julius Mayer, determined that living systems conform to basic laws of physics, most notably the first law of thermodynamics. This precept states that energy can be neither created nor destroyed but can only change forms. It explains how metabolism can transform food energy into heat energy, the chemical energy of bio-synthesis, the electrical energy of nerve action, or the mechanical energy of muscle work. If not used for such immediate purposes, food energy can be stored in the body as fat or, to a lesser extent, glycogen, the storage form of carbohydrate in liver and muscles.

According to the first law of thermodynamics, burning a food in the presence of oxygen should produce the same amount of heat as metabolism does in the body. Knowing this, scientists began to develop "bomb" calorimeters to measure the energy value of a thoroughly burned food. By the mid-1800s, they were also able to build whole-body calorimeters large enough to measure energy intake and output in larger and larger animals, eventually including sheep, horses, cows, and people. We explain how such calorimeters work in chapters 3 and 4.

THE MODERN ERA: W. O. ATWATER

Writing a book about calories required us to read a great deal of the prodigious output of Wilbur O. Atwater (1844–1907), rightfully honored as the father of modern nutrition science in the United States. Atwater studied agricultural chemistry, earned his doctorate by analyzing the chemical composition of corn, and established a food analysis laboratory at Wesleyan University.[9] In the early 1880s he traveled to Germany, where he learned how to use large, whole-body calorimeters to perform energy balance studies in humans.

On his return, Atwater continued to analyze the content of calories and nutrients in foods, based either on the amounts of heat they produced in a calorimeter or on calculations of the number of calories stored in their proteins, fats, and carbohydrates. In 1887 he summarized what was then known about food calories in a series of popular articles in *Century* magazine. There he explained that a gram of protein or carbohydrate yields less than half the energy of a gram of fat and that these differences—and variations in water content—account for variations in food calories. Most food energy, Atwater explained, is "used for the interior work of the body, breathing, keeping the blood in circulation, digestion, etc., but a large part of this is transformed into heat before it leaves the body."[10]

These conclusions were new to the public, and the *Century* articles made Atwater the most famous scientist in America. He soon held three jobs in three different cities: professor at Wesleyan in Middletown, Connecticut; director of the U.S. Department of Agriculture (USDA) Experiment Station at Storrs, Connecticut; and director of the USDA Office of Experiment Stations in Washington, DC. In these positions he continued his research on the nutrient and calorie content of foods, the ways calories are used in the body, and the calorie needs of people of different occupations and social classes. We discuss his discoveries in each of these areas in subsequent chapters.

In 1894 Atwater summarized the essence of nutritional energetics: "energy from the sun is stored in the protein and fats and carbohydrates of food, and . . . is transmuted into the heat that warms our bodies and into strength for our work and thought."[11] Three years later, in a stunning monograph of more than four hundred pages, Atwater and a colleague did what we might now call a meta-analysis of the thousands of metabolic studies that they or previous investigators had published to date. They reported their conclusions in Hippocrates-like aphorisms:

- ✦ "The animal organism requires food for a twofold purpose, (1) to furnish material for the building and repair of tissue, and (2) to supply fuel for the production of heat and energy. In serving as fuel, food protects the material of the body from consumption."
- ✦ "The food of animals consists of the so-called nutrients—protein, fat, and carbohydrates, various mineral salts, and water." (Vitamins were presumed to exist at the time but were not identified until after 1910.)
- ✦ "Food is to the body what fuel is to the fire."[12]

THE POLITICS OF CALORIE HISTORY

Atwater stated repeatedly that the purpose of his experiments was to devise the most economical diets that could meet the nutritional needs of people of various ages, occupations, and social classes. As a USDA official explained in a letter introducing one of Atwater's studies, "The immediate purpose in conducting an inquiry into the food of the colored population of the Southern States was to obtain information as to the kinds, amounts, and composition of the food materials used. The ulterior purpose was to get light upon the hygienic and pecuniary economy of their diet, its deficiencies, the ways in which it might be improved, and the steps which should be taken to bring about an improvement."[13]

We mention the USDA's goals at this point because Atwater's work has been sharply criticized for its subsequent effects on society. The science studies scholar Jessica Mudry charges that Atwater's work created an unfortunate "discourse of quantification." In her view, measuring calories caused them to be transformed "from a unit of physical science, to a unit of human fodder, and finally, through Atwater's application, a determinant of quality." By treating food components as things that could be calculated and measured, Atwater's work led to "the belief that science and quantification can tell us all that we need to know about food and eating." Instead, Mudry argues, "Any rhetoric of food and eating is incomplete and inadequate if it does not take culture, geography, tradition, experience, and taste into consideration along with the nutritional composition of foods and health," a statement with which we wholeheartedly agree.[14]

A more specific critique of Atwater's calorie investigations comes from the historian Nick Cullather. He argues that measuring calories not only takes food out of its taste and cultural traditions, but also turns food into an instrument of social control by governments. Once governments determine the number of calories needed by a population, they can quantify dietary adequacy and assume that when calories are adequate, food intake and nutritional status must also be adequate. The calorie, he says, "has never been a neutral objective measure of the contents of the dinner plate. From the first its purpose was to render food and the eating habits of populations politically legible."[15]

Atwater had said that the purpose of determining the number of calories needed by workingmen and by the "Negro" in Alabama was to establish "scientific standards of living." But Cullather argues that such standards could be and were used by governments and manufacturers to "contain wage levels while maintaining a healthy, contented workforce." He also maintains that using calorie requirements as the basis for assessing a population's need for food aid is a tool for international political domination. In making such arguments, Cullather appears to view setting standards for calorie intake as a metaphor for the mixed motivations and sometimes negative consequences associated with attempts to evaluate and meet the food requirements of undernourished populations—issues we address in later chapters.

Although we suspect that neither Mudry nor Cullather intended their analyses to be anti-scientific, their arguments appear that way to us. Should scientists not measure anything having to do with human physiology? Objections to the quantification of human energy requirements would also seem to apply to setting dietary standards for intake of protein, vitamins, and minerals, or to measurements of body weight, blood pressure, or blood sugar. Although the argument could be made that such tests are equally reductive in the sense that they reduce the health of a whole person to a single number, surely such numbers can be useful when put in context and interpreted appropriately.

We enjoy conspiracy theories as much as anyone, but we have a hard time believing that Atwater—or Lavoisier, for that matter—investigated energy metabolism out of a desire for political domination. We view both as intensely curious and committed scientists who valued knowledge for its own sake and assumed that their work would add to human knowledge and be useful. We doubt that either gave much thought to how his work might be interpreted or used by others. As we discuss in chapter 14, the humanitarian goals of many international aid agencies necessarily require some means of quantifying human food needs, and establishing standards for calorie intake can be a useful way to do this. Mudry's and Cullather's critiques, thought-provoking as they are, do not provide meaningful alternatives. They do, however, reinforce one of the central themes of this book: calories have political dimensions.

CHAPTER 3

Foods

How Scientists Count the Calories

Because the energy stored in food molecules is the same whether they are oxidized inside or outside the body, scientists can measure the energy value of a particular food to the body by burning it to completion. Nineteenth-century scientists developed calorimeters to measure the total energy stored in foods and in each of their energy-producing molecules: protein, fat, carbohydrate, and alcohol. Note again that cholesterol, vitamins, antioxidants, minerals, and water are not sources of calories. Cholesterol is excreted in bile and not metabolized. Vitamins and antioxidants are present in such small amounts—milligrams or micrograms—that they produce too little energy to bother measuring. Minerals do not store energy, and neither does water.

The device typically used to measure the energy value of food and food molecules is called a bomb calorimeter. Figure 3 shows how one of these gadgets works.[1] You place a weighed portion of food in the bomb (a sealed chamber), which has been filled with pure oxygen under high pressure. After immersing the bomb in a measured quantity of water, you ignite the food and let it burn (oxidize) to completion. The heat released by the burning warms the surrounding water. You calculate the calories from the measured rise in water temperature. Calibrated appropriately, bomb calorimeters can give quite accurate measurements of the number of calories in a food.

Bomb calorimeters work well for measuring the total number of calories in a food—its *potential* energy. But human bodies are not calorimeters. In living bodies, some of the calories in foods are lost or wasted. To determine the number of food calories that are available to the body, you have to cor-

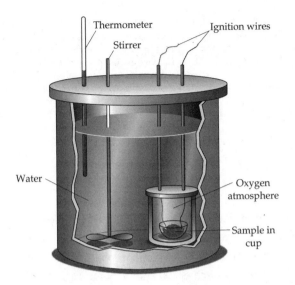

FIGURE 3. A bomb calorimeter for measuring food calories.
Food in the steel chamber (bomb) is ignited and burned
(oxidized) to completion. Calories are calculated from the
heat transferred to the surrounding water. Source: McMurry
and Fay, 2003: figure 8.9 (see note 1).

rect bomb calorimeter values for these losses. Losses occur mainly in three
ways: excretion in urine, excretion in feces due to incomplete digestion, and
inefficient metabolism. Some losses also occur in sweat, but these are usually
minor. In this chapter we discuss the first two. Chapter 7 deals with the more
complicated heat losses of metabolism.

CALORIE LOSSES: URINE

Fat and carbohydrate molecules are constructed from carbon, hydrogen, and
oxygen. In the bomb calorimeter—and in the body—fats and carbohydrates
are completely oxidized to carbon dioxide and water. So are alcohol calories,
which we reserve for their own discussion in chapter 11. Proteins, however,
are not completely oxidized to carbon dioxide and water, even though they
too are made of carbon, hydrogen, and oxygen. Proteins also contain another
element not present in carbohydrates or fats: nitrogen.

A bomb calorimeter has no problem with nitrogen. It oxidizes nitrogen
along with everything else. But in the body, metabolism converts any unused

TABLE 2   MAX RUBNER'S BOMB CALORIMETER ENERGY
VALUES FOR PROTEIN, FAT, AND CARBOHYDRATE

Food component	Calories/gram from bomb calorimeter	Calories/gram, corrected for urinary nitrogen losses
Protein	5.5	4.1
Fat	9.3	9.3
Carbohydrate	4.1	4.1

SOURCE: Atwater presents this table in his 1887 *Century* article (see note 2).

protein nitrogen into urea and other small nitrogen-containing molecules. These molecules are excreted in urine, and their calories are lost to the body.

In the nineteenth century the German physiologist Max Rubner measured the calories in proteins, fats, and carbohydrates. He knew that if he wanted to relate the calories measured in bomb calorimeters to those used in the human body, he would have to correct his results for the calories lost through nitrogen excretion. He performed experiments to determine the size of the correction. We summarize his findings in table 2.[2]

CALORIE LOSSES: INCOMPLETE DIGESTION

Rubner understood that incomplete digestion of food components reduces the calories available to the body, but he did not have the equipment or methods to develop more accurate correction factors. A decade later, Wilbur Atwater picked up where Rubner left off and attacked the digestion problem in a series of experiments remarkable for their meticulous design, conduct, and interpretation.

Reading Atwater's publications is an inspiring experience. He was a careful investigator who made impressive use of the equipment and techniques available in the late nineteenth century. His accounts of his work readily explain why he is considered the first modern nutrition scientist. Atwater based his determinations of calorie values on many different kinds of studies drawn from his own work as well as from international investigations. These included, among others:

  ✦ chemical analyses of the amount of water, protein, fat, and carbohydrate in more than 4,000 foods

TABLE 3   ATWATER'S CORRECTIONS TO BOMB CALORIMETER VALUES
FOR PROTEIN, FAT, AND CARBOHYDRATE

Food component	Bomb calorimeter value (calories/gram)	Corrected for nitrogen losses (calories/gram)	Digestibility	Corrected for availability: Atwater Values (calories/gram)
Protein	5.65	4.4	92 percent	4.0
Fat	9.4	9.4	95 percent	8.9
Carbohydrate	4.1	4.1	97 percent	4.0

SOURCE: Adapted from table 12 in Atwater and Bryant, 1900 (see note 3).

+ analyses of 185 food intake studies to estimate the average composition of diets consumed by people of different social classes, ages, and occupations

+ estimation of the digestibility of calories from protein, fat, and carbohydrate in typical mixed diets (those containing combinations of different foods)

+ bomb calorimeter measurements of the calories in foods, food components, feces, and urine

+ comparisons of calculated calorie values with those obtained in whole-body calorimeter experiments with human subjects

To determine digestibility, Atwater used a bomb calorimeter to measure the fuel value of fats, carbohydrates, and proteins. He subtracted the energy excreted in feces from the total amounts in food. As Rubner had done, Atwater corrected the calorie values obtained in protein determinations for losses of nitrogen in urine.

In 1899 Atwater (and his colleague Arthur Bryant) published calorie values for protein (4 calories per gram), fat (8.9), and carbohydrate (4). These differed from Rubner's values in that they accounted for losses in digestion.[3] Atwater's calorie numbers, corrected for losses in feces and urine, came to be known as Atwater Values. Table 3 summarizes how he arrived at them.

Atwater's bomb calorimeter was more accurate than Rubner's and yielded slightly higher values, even when corrected for nitrogen losses in urine. Atwater's experiments revealed that most of the foods he studied were almost completely digested and absorbed by the body. Only a small percentage of food proteins, fats, and carbohydrates remained undigested and were excreted in feces.

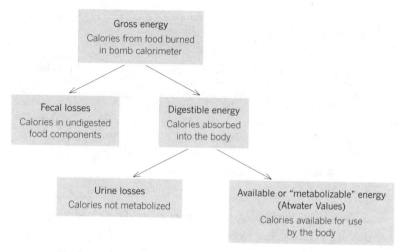

FIGURE 4. The fate of food calories in the body. Atwater Values refer to calories available to the body after subtracting those lost through incomplete digestion and excretion in feces and urine.

Atwater could use his values to predict the number of calories people ate in a day as determined through dietary records. His estimates of the number of daily calories consumed came quite close to the number of calories people used, as determined in whole-body calorimeter experiments. The difference rarely exceeded 1 percent, something that today seems unimaginable (as we later explain). Because this observed difference was so small, Atwater could safely estimate the energy value of food by assuming that proteins and carbohydrates produced 4 calories per gram and fats produced 8.9. In 1910, three years after his death, the USDA revised the Atwater Values by rounding off the calories from fat to 9 per gram.[4] As we discuss in the next section, despite numerous attempts to refine and correct the 4, 9, 4 Atwater Values, the numbers have held their own over time and continue to serve many useful purposes.

Atwater's experiments clearly distinguished the amounts of food energy available at various stages of digestion, absorption, and metabolism. These stages, which are known by different names, are illustrated in figure 4.

- *Gross energy:* the amount obtained from burning foods in a bomb calorimeter
- *Digestible energy:* the amount available to the body after subtracting fecal losses

♦ *Available or "metabolizable" energy—Atwater Values:* the amount remaining after further subtracting losses of energy in urine

Atwater Values represent available energy, or as scientists now call it, metabolizable energy—the energy from food that is available to metabolism. Available (or metabolizable) energy does correct for losses of undigested and excreted food calories. But it does *not* correct for the calories lost through dissipation of heat during metabolism, a matter we deal with in chapter 7.

ATTEMPTS TO CORRECT ATWATER VALUES

Atwater intended the values of 4, 8.9, and 4 to apply to the energy available from proteins, fats, and carbohydrates in typical foods and average diets consumed in the United States in his time. In experiments to measure the actual digestibility of specific foods, he found that some were more completely digested than others and that digestibility introduced variations in the total amount of energy available from protein, fat, and carbohydrate.

He and others did countless studies to improve the accuracy of his calorie measurements. Eventually, Atwater was able to show that the available energy from the proteins in meats, eggs, and dairy products varied from 4.25 to 4.35 calories per gram, whereas the protein calories in cereals, legumes, vegetables, and fruits varied from 2.9 to 3.7 per gram. These differences are large and might be expected to introduce significant errors in estimations of total calorie intake. But people do not usually eat only one kind of food at a meal. Most eat *mixed* diets containing several different foods. When Atwater measured the protein calories from mixed meals, he found them to average around 4 per gram, close enough to his predicted value.

Maynard's Specific Values

Because individual foods produce different energy values, Leonard Maynard, a professor at Cornell, thought Atwater Values needed improvement. In 1944 he published a critique based on individual variations among foods.[5] These variations, Maynard said, might end up causing significant errors in estimations of calorie intake. Even though Maynard's corrections were small, he wanted Atwater Values to be replaced with what he called Specific Values, numbers that considered the digestibility and availability of calories from *specific* foods. Table 4 gives some of Maynard's values. Some are lower, some

TABLE 4　SELECTED EXAMPLES OF MAYNARD'S 1944
SPECIFIC VALUES, CALORIES PER GRAM

Food	Protein	Fat	Carbohydrate
Meats	4.25	9.0	3.8
Cereals	3.7	8.35	4.1
Legumes, nuts	3.2	8.35	4.0
Fruits	3.15	8.35	3.6
Vegetables	2.9	8.35	4.0

SOURCE: Maynard, 1944 (see note 5).

are higher, and some are the same as Atwater's rounded-off 4, 9, 4 calories per gram.

USDA's Modified Atwater Values

In the years following Maynard's analysis, USDA nutritionists and chemists took his criticisms to heart and developed better methods for analyzing the energy and nutrient content of foods. In 1955 they published a state-of-the-art review of the history and accuracy of calorie determinations, in which they analyzed human experiments quantifying the digestibility of food plants dating back to 1875. The review provided detailed explanations of the methods used to update Atwater's and Maynard's figures and to test the accuracy of their proposed Modified Atwater Values. USDA staff published a "slightly revised" version of this review in 1973. We put this in quotation marks because, despite much searching, we are unable to find any difference between the two publications other than the addition of a brief preface to the 1973 edition.[6] We give some examples of USDA Modified Atwater Values in table 5.

To test the modified values, USDA investigators conducted more than one hundred experiments with human volunteers who were asked to consume diets of widely varying—*wildly* may be a better word—food composition. The diets seem quite odd, even considering that they were apparently designed for extreme variations in intake of one food group or another. To pick a particularly unusual example: one of the daily diets in the fruit-and-nut category consisted of four pounds of persimmons, half a pound of peanuts, an ounce of wheat cereal, two ounces of milk, a tablespoon of tomatoes, and two teaspoons of olive oil.[7]

TABLE 5   SELECTED EXAMPLES OF 1955 USDA MODIFIED
ATWATER VALUES, CALORIES PER GRAM

Food	Protein	Fat	Carbohydrate
Meat and fish	4.27	9.02	—
Milk products	4.27	8.79	3.87
Fruits, most	3.36	8.37	3.60
Pasta	3.91	8.37	4.12
Peas and beans	3.47	8.37	4.07
Vegetables, most	2.44	8.37	3.57
Sugar	—	—	3.87

SOURCE: Merrill and Watt, 1955 (see note 6).

To determine the available calories in such diets, USDA scientists burned the foods in a bomb calorimeter. They collected feces and urine from the volunteers who ate the foods, then burned the excretion products in the calorimeter. After counting the food calories and subtracting the calories in the excretion products, they concluded that the persimmon-peanut diet provided 2,399 calories per day.

For this same diet, USDA investigators also measured the amount of protein, fat, and carbohydrate in each food (perhaps explaining why the experimental diets contained so few foods). They calculated the calories using Atwater Values and Modified Atwater Values. The modified values gave the total calories as 2,406, only 7 calories higher than the value obtained in the feeding experiment. In contrast, the Atwater Values gave 2,622. For this unusual and minimally varied high-fiber diet, the result using Atwater Values was about 9 percent higher than those determined experimentally. This was at the extreme of variation. For most of the diets tested, the experimental and calculated methods produced results that differed by an average of about 2 percent, and the variation rarely exceeded 5 percent. Whether variations in this range make any difference to body weight is a question we return to in later chapters.

Because the results using Modified Atwater Values were comparable to those obtained from human digestion experiments, USDA scientists concluded that the modified values should be used until further research indicated a need for change. In the subsequent half century, no such need has emerged, apparently. The 1955 Modified Atwater Values are still the basis of USDA food composition data, as we discuss in chapter 10.

The Life Science Research Office Evaluation

In 1983 the Life Science Research Office (LSRO) of the Federation of American Societies for Experimental Biology decided to evaluate whether Atwater Values should remain the basis for calories listed in the USDA's food composition tables.[8] After weighing the strengths and limitations of Atwater Values, the LSRO investigators concluded that "the Atwater System provides estimates of metabolizable energy within the limits of accuracy in measuring food intake and also within the predictive limits of food composition tables." Translation: they considered Atwater Values good enough to use for most practical purposes, given the many other sources of error that affect determinations of calorie intake and food composition. The LSRO agreed that improving the Atwater Values in any biologically meaningful way would require much better data on food composition and on the digestibility of a much greater range of food products.

IMPLICATIONS

Because no subsequent investigation has produced calorie numbers that improve the definition of metabolizable energy in any meaningful way, the 4, 9, 4 Atwater Values remain in active use. If you know the grams of sugar—a carbohydrate—in your soda or lollipop, you can estimate the number of calories it contains by multiplying grams by 4. If you want to estimate the calories in your daily diet, you can list the foods, find out how many grams of protein, fat, and carbohydrate each contains, and multiply the totals by 4, 9, and 4, respectively.

More than one hundred years after Atwater's death, Atwater Values can still be seen at the bottom of some food package labels. In part because Atwater Values are approximations, the FDA allows the food industry considerable leeway in calculating the calorie content of packaged foods and items listed on restaurant menu boards.[9] As we discuss further in chapter 23, they may determine the calories in their products by using:

+ Atwater Values, 4, 9, 4
+ the USDA's 1955 Modified Atwater Values as "updated" in 1973
+ Atwater Values further corrected for undigested fiber

- values established or approved by the FDA for specific foods or ingredients
- bomb calorimetry figures corrected for loss of urinary nitrogen

These methods produce varying results, but all give close enough estimates of calorie content. All, it should be evident, are likely to be inaccurate to some degree, not least because none of them accounts for the heat losses that occur during metabolism. We defer consideration of those heat losses to chapter 7 because a discussion about them requires an explanation of how such things are measured. That explanation comes next.

CHAPTER 4

Bodies

How Scientists Measure the Use of Calories

Nineteenth-century scientists were eager to find out how many calories someone might need to maintain basic body functions, activities, and weight. To do so, they had to be able to measure the amounts of heat produced when people were engaged in daily activities. They started by inventing devices—calorimeters—to measure the heat produced by small animals. Later they figured out how to construct calorimeters large enough to house people and farm animals. These "whole-body" calorimeters allowed them to make *direct* measurements of heat output.

Studies using even the largest calorimeters required people to be confined to the device, and space considerations limited what study subjects could be asked to do. Scientists wanted to develop less physically restrictive methods to measure the use of calories *indirectly*. They figured out two ways to do this. They could calculate calories from measurements either of the amount of oxygen breathed in and "burned" in the body or of the differential rates of disappearance of certain chemicals from the body. These methods produce results that are similar to those obtained using whole-body calorimeters. Today indirect methods are employed most often to measure the use—the expenditure—of calories by the body.

In this chapter we focus on the principal methods for measuring the ways calories are used in the human body. We describe the methods at this point because so much of what follows depends on understanding what, exactly, scientists are measuring. A constant theme of this book is the distinction between the numbers obtained by *measuring* the calories in foods or used by the body as compared to the numbers obtained by various means of *estimation*. To decide whether this distinction makes any real difference, it helps to know something about what the methods measure and how they work.

DIRECT WHOLE-BODY CALORIMETRY: MEASURING HEAT PRODUCTION

In the late eighteenth century, as we noted earlier, the French scientist Antoine Lavoisier built one of the first whole-body calorimeters capable of directly measuring the heat produced by a small animal—a guinea pig. Figure 5 illustrates the design of his device.

Lavoisier placed the guinea pig in the interior chamber of the double-walled container, surrounded the chamber with ice, and measured the amount of water produced as the ice melted. He filled the outer jacket of the device with ice and water to prevent ambient heat from melting the ice in the inner chamber. Scientists of his era already knew how much heat was needed to melt ice.[1] Knowing that, Lavoisier could calculate the amount of heat produced by his enclosed guinea pig.

In the 1860s European scientists began to build more sophisticated calorimeters, large enough to house people. Wilbur Atwater went to Europe to work with some of the researchers who had constructed these devices. When he returned to the United States he obtained funding to build his own. By 1895 he had built what was then a state-of-the-art calorimeter at Wesleyan University that was able to house a human volunteer for days at a time. Figure 6 shows the calorimeter, which worked on the same principle as Lavoisier's. Its chamber was surrounded by walls filled with circulating water. Atwater could measure the heat produced by a person living in the chamber by the rise in temperature of the surrounding water.

In 1897 Atwater and his colleagues wrote lengthy and detailed descriptions of their calorimeter studies, in which they pointed out that "The occupants of the chamber passed the time in such ways as were in general most agreeable under the circumstances. They observed regular hours of eating and sleeping. . . . Abundant opportunity was given for reading, considerable conversation was held between the occupant and the men who did the work outside, and the monotony was also relieved from time to time by visitors."[2]

We can debate just how agreeable such studies might have been to endure, but there is no question that they yielded highly accurate measurements.

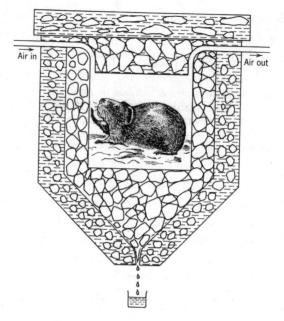

FIGURE 5. Antoine Lavoisier's calorimeter. This device was large enough to measure the heat generated by a guinea pig. Source: Kleiber, 1961 (see note 7).

Over periods of several days, Atwater could directly measure—and accurately account for—the calories in the food the subjects ate and in those they excreted in urine and feces, stored in their bodies, and expended as heat. He had constructed the calorimeter in a way that allowed him to measure the amounts of oxygen his study subjects inhaled and the amounts of carbon dioxide they exhaled, meaning that he could use the device to calculate calories directly from heat but also indirectly from measurements of the components of air breathed in and out. To do all this, Atwater had to develop careful and reproducible methods for using the calorimeter, for measuring oxygen and carbon dioxide, and for analyzing the energy content of food, feces, and urine.

A few years later Henry Armsby built an even larger calorimeter at Pennsylvania State College, to enable studies of the metabolism—and, ultimately, food needs—of farm animals. This calorimeter could also measure heat production indirectly as well as directly. Considered a marvel of technology in 1902, Armsby's laboratory was the size of a small New York City apartment, and the calorimeter chamber alone could accommodate a large cow or draft

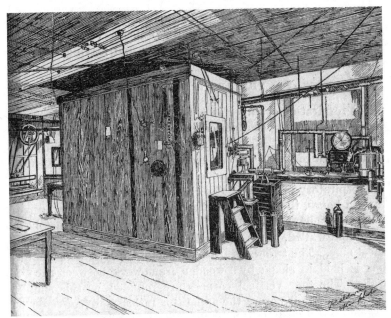

FIGURE 6. Wilbur Atwater's whole-body calorimeter for measuring calorie input and output in human volunteers. Someone could live in this device for days at a time while Atwater and his colleagues measured everything the volunteer ate, drank, excreted, and breathed. Source: Atwater, Woods, and Benedict, 1897 (see note 2).

horse. Armsby's successors rebuilt the calorimeter to handle four sheep at a time in the 1940s and modified it again in the 1950s to house human subjects. But by that time the technology had moved on. The university converted the building to a museum in 1969, open by appointment.

We arranged to see the museum on a visit to Penn State and noted that it is marked by a plaque: "Designed and first operated in 1902 by pioneer animal nutritionist Henry Armsby, the calorimeter was housed in this specially constructed building and monitored an animal's metabolism to determine the net energy value of food—the portion of food energy that an animal used to produce milk or meat. It attracted worldwide scientific interest and helped to develop feeds of higher nutritive value."[3]

In the 1950s T. H. Benzinger developed a "gradient layer" calorimeter. Instead of using surrounding water to absorb the heat, this calorimeter had sensors that measured the passage of heat through its walls.[4] In modern calorimeter chambers, human subjects can live and carry out relatively normal activities for days in reasonable, although somewhat claustrophobic, comfort.

INDIRECT CALORIMETRY: MEASURING
OXYGEN AND CARBON DIOXIDE

The calorimeters of Lavoisier, Atwater, and Armsby were *direct* calorimeters. They could be used to measure the amount of heat required to melt ice or warm water. Atwater's and Armsby's calorimeters also measured heat production *indirectly*—through the amounts of oxygen breathed in and used and of carbon dioxide given off by the animal or person enclosed in the chamber. In the 1970s and 1980s, scientists built indirect, room-size, whole-body "respiration" calorimeters that measured only oxygen intake and carbon dioxide "excretion." They used these calorimeters to study energy metabolism and the energy cost of various activities under tightly controlled conditions. The respiration calorimeter at the USDA experiment station at Beltsville, Maryland, for example, has a floor area of ninety square feet furnished with a bed, desk, chair, sink, toilet, lamps, audio speakers, and exercise equipment. The USDA Human Nutrition Center at Baylor University operates four room-size indirect calorimeters designed to measure energy use over periods ranging from minutes to twenty-four hours.[5]

If you are housed in one of these chambers, scientists can estimate the number of calories you require from the amount of oxygen you breathe in and use.[6] They are able to do this because the amount of heat you emit is proportional to the amount of oxygen you "consume." Consider, for example, how hard you have to breathe when running up stairs. Air is about 20 percent oxygen—the rest is mostly nitrogen. Scientists measure oxygen in liters (roughly equivalent to quarts). A liter of pure oxygen—not air—that you breathe in and use corresponds to an energy output of about 5 calories. You inhale and use more oxygen when your activity is more intense.

But because even the best of whole-body respiration calorimeters requires people to be confined, the devices cannot be used to measure energy expenditure during activities such as running, playing sports, swimming, or anything else that requires more space. As early as the 1890s, scientists knew that they needed some less restrictive way to measure energy use, and they invented portable indirect calorimeters to measure oxygen uptake. These devices had immediate uses in medicine. Physicians could take the portable devices to hospitals and measure the calorie needs of patients at the bedside. Over the years, scientists refined these indirect calorimeters, and many are now small enough to be used during almost any imaginable physical activity.

CORRECTING FOR THE "FUEL" MIX

Five calories per liter of oxygen used in the body is an estimate, not a precise figure. The number of calories you expend per liter of oxygen turns out to depend on what you have been eating. To obtain more accurate values for calorie expenditure, scientists have to correct for the "fuel"—the mix of proteins, fats, and carbohydrates—that you are metabolizing at any given moment.

Because of their particular molecular configurations, pure proteins, fats, and carbohydrates release different amounts of heat per liter of oxygen consumed. Scientists have measured these amounts and know them quite precisely: protein and fat release 4.7 calories per liter of oxygen, and carbohydrate releases 5. The difference between 4.7 and 5 is not great, but it can add up to 100 calories or more in people who consume 400 to 500 liters of oxygen a day, which most people do.

Although these numbers look something like Atwater Values, they are entirely different. Atwater Values refer to calories *per gram* of protein, fat, or carbohydrate in food. The numbers here are calories *per liter* of oxygen used in the body. They were calculated by completely oxidizing food molecules, measuring the total heat given off (gross energy), and dividing this by the number of liters of oxygen used in the process.

But except for things like sugar and salad oil, you do not usually eat pure carbohydrate or fat. You eat foods containing varying proportions of protein, fat, and carbohydrate. If you think this must mean that your ratio of carbon dioxide to oxygen varies throughout the day depending on what you just ate, you are quite right. Researchers must correct calories per liter of oxygen for differences in the ratio of exhaled carbon dioxide to inhaled oxygen over time. This ratio has its own name: the respiratory quotient (RQ). If you would like to know more about how it is determined, see appendix 2.

When measurements do not need to be precise, scientists can simply count the liters of oxygen used and multiply that by a factor of 5 or, somewhat more accurately, 4.8, to come up with the number of calories used. Either way, the result is unlikely to differ by more than 5 percent from the more accurately measured and corrected values. Although a 5 percent difference may seem worth worrying about, it turns out to be small relative to the much larger variations in the calories you consume and expend.

Another way to estimate calorie use by indirect calorimetry is to measure the amount of carbon dioxide breathed out. This too depends on what you just ate. The number of calories produced per liter of exhaled carbon dioxide is 6.6 when fat is the fuel, 5.6 when it is protein, and 5.0 when it is carbohydrate.[7] The figure for mixed diets is something in between. These distinctions do make a difference in calorie calculations derived from the most important of the indirect measurement methods: doubly labeled water.

INDIRECT CALORIMETRY: DOUBLY LABELED WATER

The doubly labeled water method for determining calorie expenditure is so accurate that it is currently considered the gold standard for such determinations. The method was devised in the 1960s as a way to measure the number of calories used at rest and in free, unrestricted physical activity. In effect, doubly labeled water is a chemical method for measuring the amount of exhaled carbon dioxide (CO_2 in chemical designation). For years, scientists used this method to study energy production in small animals, but the high cost of the isotopes made it too expensive for use with larger animals or people. As soon as the price of the isotopes dropped to reasonable levels, researchers began using them to study human energy expenditure.[8]

Doubly labeled water uses nonradioactive stable isotopes—naturally occurring alternative forms—of hydrogen and oxygen to figure out how much CO_2 is exhaled over time. The method uses two distinct forms of water labeled with these isotopes. Normally, water—identified chemically as H_2O—consists of two atoms of hydrogen (atomic weight 1) and one of oxygen (atomic weight 16). *Doubly labeled* refers to two forms of water containing isotopes:

+ heavy-hydrogen (deuterium) water, designated ^2H_2O and enriched with the deuterium isotope of hydrogen (^2H), which has an atomic weight of 2 rather than 1

+ heavy-oxygen water, designated $H_2^{18}O$ and enriched with oxygen of atomic weight 18 (hence: ^{18}O) rather than 16

If you volunteer to participate in a doubly labeled water experiment, here is what happens. You drink water containing measured amounts of the two isotopes. The isotopes mix with all the water in your body. After a good night's sleep, you report back to the lab and donate a urine sample. Technicians measure the levels of the isotopes in a sample of your urine using appropriate analytical equipment. During the two or three weeks of the experiment, you continue to excrete water in the usual way through urine, sweat, and your moist breath. You will also excrete the isotopes in that water. As you replace the water by your usual drinking and eating, the isotopes in your body become increasingly diluted. At the end of the experiment you donate another urine sample, and technicians measure how much of each isotope is left.[9]

The key to the doubly labeled water method is that *all* of the ^2H isotope that disappears from your body will be excreted in water. But the ^{18}O isotope is lost in two ways. Some disappears in the water along with the ^2H. But some also is lost in the carbon dioxide you breathe out. This means that more ^{18}O than ^2H is excreted from your body over time. This, in turn, means that your urine will contain less ^{18}O than ^2H at the end of the experiment. From the difference between the amounts of the two isotopes in an overnight urine sample, researchers can calculate the number of liters of carbon dioxide you breathed out during the course of the experiment, as determined through the use of appropriate (albeit quite complicated) equations. Once you know the number of liters of carbon dioxide, you can convert it to calories by multiplying by the appropriate conversion factors corrected for the RQ.

Doubly labeled water experiments usually last two to three weeks, periods long enough to allow day-to-day deviations in calorie use to be averaged out. When corrected for the RQ, such studies can produce results that are within 2 percent of whole-body calorimetry measurements of carbon dioxide production. Because isotope methods do not require people to be confined in calorimeters or to carry or be attached to oxygen-uptake devices, doubly labeled water techniques are now commonly used for examining energy expenditure in people going about their daily activities. The studies usually are done on relatively small numbers of people at a time, mainly for reasons of cost and logistics, but by now many people have had their energy expenditure measured by this method.[10] In chapter 9 we show how such measurements have been used to estimate the total energy expenditure of men and women of various ages and body weights.

This chapter covered methods for *measuring* calorie use, not estimating it. This is an important distinction. Even with sources of error, measurements of calorie intake and expenditure are far more accurate than estimations. Keep this point in mind when considering how calories work in the body, the question to which we now turn.

PART TWO

Why You Need Calories
Survival, Warmth, and Work

We devoted earlier chapters to the number of calories in proteins, fats, and carbohydrates; the number of calories from these components in foods used by the body; and the ways scientists arrived at those numbers. We did this to emphasize that scientists can accurately measure calories in food or the body, but doing so requires complicated laboratory equipment such as bomb or whole-body calorimeters or chemical techniques that require isotopes and expensive machines. For convenience, it is much easier to estimate calorie numbers using indirect measurements or calculations. Although calorie estimates are grounded in experiment, some aspects of the use of calories by the body are extremely difficult to measure.

Consider your own diet for a moment. You almost certainly eat varying amounts of different kinds of foods each day. The human body will digest, absorb, metabolize, and excrete those foods or their metabolic products in a more or less predictable way, with some variation among individuals. Small losses of energy occur at every stage of digestion, absorption, and metabolism. The size of these losses depends on matters such as the amount of fiber the foods provide; the relative proportions of protein, fat, and carbohydrate in the foods; and how available these components are to digestive enzymes.

In this part of the book we discuss how the digestion, absorption, and metabolism of food molecules make energy available to the body. We also review how bodies use this energy to maintain basic life functions, stay warm, and be active. Metabolism, as we explain here, is designed to convert the substances you get from food—any food, no matter whether derived from animals or plants—into your own body parts while at the same time providing the energy you need to conduct your daily life. Understanding metabolism is good preparation for our later discussions of the number of calories you might need to support your basic body functions, keep yourself warm, and fuel whatever activities you happen to be doing.

CHAPTER 5

Metabolism

How the Body Turns Food into Energy

Our colleagues in anthropology are fond of saying "You are what you eat." By this they mean that food choices reveal a great deal about your position in society—age, family background, educational level, religion, and other such things. If you know what people eat, you can make some pretty good guesses about where they come from, what they believe, and how educated and rich or poor they are. Food choices also differ in the ways they affect health. But the digestive tract makes few such distinctions. Unless you have a genetic or acquired intolerance to certain foods, your digestive enzymes are going to process whatever energy-yielding food components get into your digestive tract in exactly the same way they do in other animals and people.[1]

Because of this universality, people can survive on diets of extraordinary diversity in the type and composition of food. From the standpoint of calories, digestion is concerned only with proteins, fats, and carbohydrates. Alcohol is not digested; it is absorbed intact. Because of the way digestion works, your diet can vary from day to day in the foods you eat and their amounts. The principle of digestion is elegant in biological terms. Digestion converts proteins, fats, and carbohydrates uniquely characteristic of the particular food plant or animal you are eating into subunits that are common to all proteins, fats, and carbohydrates, yours included. You can use the subunits to build your own body parts or to provide energy.

Food proteins, fats, and carbohydrates are highly ordered, complex structures that are entirely specific to the plant or animal food from which they derive. Each of these energy-yielding components is constructed from subunits. In all proteins, whether in food or in you, the subunits are amino acids. In complex carbohydrates (starch), the subunits are "simple" carbohydrates, or sugars. In fats, they are fatty acids linked to glycerol, a small sugar-alcohol. Usually, three fatty acids link to glycerol, which is why food and body fats are sometimes referred to as triglycerides. It takes energy to build amino acids into proteins, sugars into complex carbohydrates, and triglycerides into fat. Much of that energy is stored in the bonds that hold the subunits together in large, complex structures. During digestion, enzymes split the bonds that link the subunits, releasing a little energy. The amino acid, fatty acid, and sugar subunits are small enough to be absorbed into the body.

Metabolism uses enzymes to break the subunits into smaller and smaller pieces, releasing even more energy. It extracts energy from the subunits through oxidation reactions—those involving oxygen—and uses the energy to power everything bodies do: transmit nerve impulses, breathe, circulate blood, excrete wastes, use muscles, and stay warm. Overall, the extraction of energy from food molecules takes place in distinct stages:

- *Digestion* disassembles the large, complex protein, fat, and carbohydrate structures that are *uniquely* characteristic of particular foods—beef, broccoli, or peanuts, for example—into amino acids, fatty acids, and simple sugars that are common to foods and to the people who eat them.

- *Absorption* brings amino acids, fatty acids, and sugars from the digestive tract into the interior of the body.

- *Excretion* gets rid of the waste products of digestion and metabolism through feces and urine.

- *Metabolism* disassembles the products of digestion into even smaller pieces or uses them to construct body tissues. Eventually, it converts whatever small pieces remain to carbon dioxide and water. Carbon dioxide is exhaled in breath. Water is excreted in urine. Throughout metabolism, the various oxidation reactions that disassemble food molecules release energy that the body can use.

DIGESTION AND ABSORPTION

Food proteins, fats, and carbohydrates are usually too large to be absorbed through the intestinal wall. They must be disassembled—digested—into

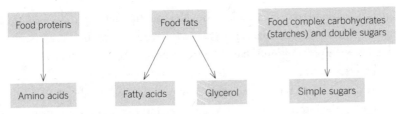

FIGURE 7. Digestion of food components. Enzymes in the mouth, stomach, and small intestine break down large molecules uniquely characteristic of specific plant and animal foods into subunits common to all living organisms. The subunits are small enough to be absorbed into the body. Digestion releases some heat energy, but the amount is small relative to amounts released during metabolism.

pieces small enough to be taken across the digestive tract and into the body. The disassembly is accomplished quite efficiently by digestive enzymes. During digestion, enzymes convert food proteins into amino acids, and food starches (complex carbohydrates) and slightly complex (double) sugars like sucrose into simple sugars such as glucose and fructose.

Digestive enzymes convert food fats (triglycerides) into fatty acids, monoglycerides, diglycerides, and glycerol, all of which can be absorbed. For simplicity, we will ignore the intermediate glycerides and assume that fats are digested to fatty acids and glycerol. We summarize these processes in figure 7.

Digestion releases some energy as heat, but the amount is so small—less than 1 percent of the calories in foods—that it usually can be ignored by everyone except researchers. The disassembly of complex food components releases very little heat and wastes few calories. The process of digestion itself also requires only small amounts of energy, mostly to construct digestive enzymes or move the products of digestion across the intestinal wall and into the body.

The fate of amino acids, fatty acids, and sugars in the body may differ depending on whether you are a child or an adult, growing or pregnant, sedentary or active. But the entire point of digestion is to take anything that was once alive and edible—plant or animal, fish or fowl—and turn its proteins, fats, and carbohydrates into amino acids, fatty acids, and sugars that you can metabolize for your own energy or to build your own tissues. The process of digestion occurs without respect to issues of culture, personal identity, socioeconomic status, or food choice. Its job is strictly to convert food—*any* food—into components that can be absorbed into your body where you can use them.

To get a sense of how the digestive tract works, we like to think of it as a tube with a very large surface area. The tube goes through the body, from the mouth at one end to the anus at the other. One function of the digestive tube is to keep the parts of food that are indigestible or too big to absorb outside the body's working metabolic area until they can be taken apart by digestive enzymes or excreted. Once the smaller molecules are absorbed across the wall of the intestinal tube, these amino acids, fatty acids, and sugars are functionally inside the body's working area, where they become available to produce energy or perform other biological tasks.

EXCRETION

Undigested and unabsorbed food materials hardly ever get across the wall of the digestive tube. They remain inside it, to be excreted as fecal matter. Whatever calories they contain are lost. But digestion, as Wilbur Atwater's experiments revealed, is a remarkably efficient process. Only small percentages of the proteins, fats, and carbohydrates in foods escape disassembly by digestive enzymes. The components that manage to escape digestion do so because they are structured too tightly or in some other way that makes them impervious to human digestive enzymes. Fiber, the collective name given to various kinds of large, indigestible carbohydrates in food plants, falls into the impervious category. So do some food proteins that are folded so tightly or inconveniently that digestive enzymes are unable to attack them.[2] And so do some artificial fats, sweeteners, and other food additives chemically constructed to resist enzyme action. Most natural fats, on the other hand, are 97 percent digested.

Atwater, Leonard Maynard, and many subsequent investigators experimentally confirmed digestive variability. They demonstrated that animal foods—meat and dairy—are quite similar and predictable in their digestibility and highly digestible whether cooked or raw. In contrast, plant foods vary greatly in digestibility, depending on their fiber composition and content, and they tend to be more completely digested when cooked. Heat breaks open the cell walls of plant foods and makes their internal components more accessible to digestive enzymes.[3]

Digestion and absorption occur mainly in the part of the digestive tube called the small intestine, despite its twenty-five-foot length. Undigested food molecules pass into the much shorter large intestine (also called the bowel or colon), an organ brimming with bacteria eager to take advantage of any food that comes their way. Intestinal bacteria are able to break apart some components of fiber.

Bacterial digestion has its own name: fermentation. This process is responsible for the gas that often accompanies the eating of foods impervious to human digestive enzymes—beans, for example. Beans contain forms of carbohydrate structured in such a way that human enzymes cannot act on them. Bacterial enzymes have no such limitations. Fermentation also creates by-products that are absorbed through the wall of the large intestine. When this happens, some of the by-product molecules can be used as sources of energy. Any food components left after bacterial digestion, along with sloughed-off intestinal cells and billions of bacteria, are excreted from the body as feces.

METABOLISM: ATP AND THE PRODUCTION OF ENERGY

Once absorbed into the body, the products of the digestion of proteins, fats, and carbohydrates—amino acids, fatty acids, and sugars—are available to be metabolized. *Metabolism* is the term given to the entire process of using the molecules in the food you eat to maintain your basic functions, build new molecules characteristic of your own body, use your muscles, and produce energy. Metabolism takes amino acids, fatty acids, and sugars and does one of three things with them:

+ produces energy by breaking them apart
+ uses energy to assemble them into new body molecules
+ uses energy to store them for later use

To produce energy, enzymes convert amino acids, fatty acids, and sugars step by step into smaller and smaller pieces, eventually to be excreted as carbon dioxide and water. Some of the energy produced in these steps is released as heat, but much of it is trapped for later use.

All living plants and animals use one particular molecule for this precise trapping purpose: adenosine triphosphate (ATP). ATP captures energy in its three phosphate bonds. The body can use the energy stored in ATP to power whatever chemical, electrical, or mechanical functions are needed. When extra energy is available, ATP is synthesized from adenosine diphosphate (ADP) and phosphate (P):[4]

$$Energy + ADP + P \rightarrow ATP$$

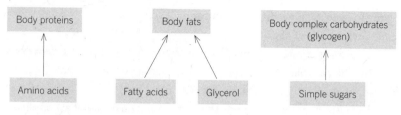

FIGURE 8. Construction of body proteins, fats, and carbohydrates from digested and absorbed or newly constructed subunits. Enzymes build body molecules using energy obtained from the conversion of ATP to ADP.

Any time the body needs energy, enzymes reverse this reaction and convert ATP to ADP and phosphate:

$$ATP \rightarrow ADP + P + energy$$

If you eat more food than you need to meet your immediate energy requirements, ATP can be used to power the construction of body fats, proteins (muscles, enzymes, skin, hair, etc.), and carbohydrates (glycogen) from their basic subunits, as shown in figure 8.

ATP also participates in all the other energy-requiring steps in metabolism: the construction of enzymes and hormones, the absorption of food molecules into the body, the transmission of nerve impulses, the action of muscles, and whatever thinking and anything else the brain needs to do.

Biological processes are never totally efficient, and metabolism is no exception. ATP cannot capture all of the potential energy stored in amino acids, fatty acids, and sugars. The complete disassembly of one molecule of the sugar glucose to carbon dioxide and water, for example, generates 36 to 38 molecules of ATP, depending on the pathway used for metabolism. But ATP molecules are able to trap only about 40 percent of this energy. The remaining 60 percent is dissipated as heat. This heat helps to maintain body temperature.

Some of the heat derives from what is called the thermic effect of food—the increase in heat production that occurs after eating—a phenomenon that we describe in chapter 7. But first we deal with basal metabolic needs, the number of calories required every day to keep body systems functioning.

CHAPTER 6

The First Use of Calories

Basic Life Functions

For years scientists have divided the use of calories in the body into three distinct compartments—basal metabolism, the heat ("thermic") effect of food, and work or physical activity. During much of the twentieth century and continuing into the twenty-first, physiologists have expended a great many of their own calories in thought and action to measure the precise number of calories used to power each of these separate compartments. In this chapter we deal with the energy cost of basic body "housekeeping" functions—the proportionately large number of calories needed to fuel the brain, heart, lungs, kidneys, nervous system, and everything else that happens automatically to keep your body alive without conscious muscle activity. Unless you engage in a great deal of physical activity, basal metabolism is likely to account for about two-thirds of your total calorie needs.

MEASURING THE BASAL METABOLIC RATE (BMR)

Nineteenth-century physiologists were impressed by how accurately they could predict the amount of heat produced in whole-body calorimeter experiments by people who were at rest, fasting, and doing no muscle work. In the 1890s the German physiologist Adolf Magnus-Levy used the term *Grundumsatz*—literally "basic rate"—to describe the heat produced in this resting-and-fasting state. Later Graham Lusk took credit for giving it the name still used in English: basal metabolism.[1] The twentieth-century nutritionist H. H. Mitchell defined *basal metabolism* as "the minimal expenditure of energy compatible with life."[2] By this, he meant the substantial amounts of energy needed to support such functions as brain activity, blood circulation, breathing, and waste removal.

Physiologists use the term *basal metabolic rate* (BMR) to refer to the exact number of calories required to support basal functions each day. The BMR is measured in calories per day, but its more accurate meaning is calories per day under highly specific and restrictive conditions. These conditions require BMR measurements to be taken under extremely precise circumstances. To have it evaluated accurately, people whose BMR is being measured must be:

+ awake
+ fasting for the previous twelve to fourteen hours (but otherwise normally nourished)
+ healthy
+ at rest
+ in a room with a comfortable ambient temperature
+ mentally tranquil

These conditions make sense if you think about it. They prevent the introduction of environmental factors or physical actions that might raise heat production over basal levels. Anything along the lines of eating, hunger, activity, sweating, shivering, and stress raises heat production.

But consider how difficult it might be for you to meet those conditions. Unless you volunteer to have your BMR measured in a whole-body calorimeter, you need to get yourself up, dressed, and to a doctor's office—activities not necessarily conducive to mental tranquility. For reasons of practicality, physiologists cut corners on the restrictions. They measure a surrogate for the BMR—the Resting Energy Expenditure (REE).

REE measurements merely require subjects to be at rest. If these people have not eaten or exercised within the previous eight hours or so, the REE value is close to the BMR and is, in fact, a quite reasonable surrogate. But when subjects are not rested and have recently been eating, the REE can be as much as 20 percent higher than the BMR, a significant error.[3] Most experiments to measure the REE control the conditions fairly carefully. When they do, the BMR and the REE can be considered equivalent enough for most purposes (there's that "good enough" phrase again). For simplicity, we will use the term BMR when discussing the results of studies that measured or estimated either the BMR or the REE.

ESTIMATING THE BMR

Because measuring either the BMR or the REE is expensive and time-consuming, scientists and medical personnel want to avoid having to do it. They had the idea that if they could work out a mathematical formula for estimating resting metabolism with reasonable accuracy, they would be able to substitute the formula for actual experiments. To develop the formula, they began with animals. This made sense because the metabolic rate of warm-blooded animals is so predictable that early investigators thought of it as a biological constant. They could see that the resting metabolism of small animals was higher than that of large animals. But the difference was not proportional to weight. Instead, it was proportional to body surface area. When scientists measured the heat produced by resting animals of any size, it turned out to be about 1,000 calories per day per square meter of body surface area, as we show in table 6.

The relationship that enables scientists to predict the BMR of living creatures of different sizes is called the Surface Area Law. Small animals have more skin surface relative to their weight than larger animals. Because skin radiates heat, it takes more calories to maintain body temperature in animals with relatively large surface areas for their body size.

But measuring the surface area of a three-dimensional body is a challenging task, one quite difficult to accomplish in practice. It is much, much easier to measure body weight. By playing around with numbers, scientists developed formulas to relate BMR to body weight. In the 1930s, for example, Max Kleiber estimated the BMR of mammals of varying sizes using a rather nonintuitive formula that must have been tedious to use in the precalculator era: BMR = 70 times the three-fourths power of body weight in kilograms.[4]

Within a given species of animal—humans, for example—BMR prediction equations can be more accurate. In 1919 Francis Benedict and his colleague J. Arthur Harris developed equations to predict the BMR of men and women based on height and body weight. We give the equations in the notes to this chapter.[5] We worked with the Harris-Benedict equations while we were in graduate school but did not find them much fun to use. Difficult

TABLE 6   HEAT PRODUCED BY RESTING ANIMALS

Animal	Body weight in kilograms (kg)	Calories per day released per kg of body weight	Calories per day released per square meter of body surface area
Horse	441.0	10	950
Pig	128.0	20	1,080
Man	64.3	30	1,040
Dog	15.2	50	1,040
Goose	3.5	70	970
Rabbit	2.5	75	780
Mouse	0.02	210	1,190

SOURCE: Adapted from Mitchell, 1962:17 (see note 2).
NOTE: A kilogram is 2.2 pounds. All calorie figures rounded off.

as they were to calculate, they did yield BMR estimates close to measured values, and they remain the standard for most such estimates to this day.

One determined effort to improve on the Harris-Benedict equations took place in the 1980s. A United Nations committee was working on establishing international standards for the daily calorie requirements of human populations. For reasons of its own, the committee decided that it wanted to express the calorie requirements as multiples of the BMR—for example, 1.5 or 2.0 times the calories required for the BMR. The size of the multiples would depend on levels of physical activity. But to use such multiples, the committee needed better data on the average BMRs of men and women of varying ages than were available at that time. To get this information, it commissioned a comprehensive review of worldwide BMR measurements.[6]

As it turned out, plenty of such measurements had been taken. The review ended up evaluating BMR measurements derived from studies of nearly 7,400 individuals during the sixty years following Harris and Benedict's work. Based on these measurements, the British physiologist W. N. Schofield was able to develop BMR formulas that were more accurate, easier to use, and more specific. His formulas, which we give in the notes, were based on body weights and heights but applied to men and women in four different age groups.[7]

Never mind the formulas. Today estimating a BMR could not be easier. If you want to find out your own BMR, you can go online and search for a website that hosts a BMR calculator. You type in your height, weight, age,

TABLE 7   BASAL METABOLIC RATE (BMR) ESTIMATED
BY FOUR METHODS, CALORIES PER DAY

Method	Marion Nestle	Malden Nesheim
Kleiber formula	1,415	2,045
Schofield formula	1,195	1,780
Harris-Benedict formula	1,135	1,700
Online BMR calculator	1,130	1,690

and sex, push the button, and there you have it—an estimate, and probably a quite reasonable one, of the calories required each day for your basic body functions. These are generally based on the Harris-Benedict equations rather than the more accurate Schofield ones, but they still give useful information.

We thought it would be instructive to calculate our own BMRs using the Kleiber, Harris-Benedict, and Schofield equations and compare them to results obtained from an online BMR calculator.[8] We summarize what we found in table 7.

The Kleiber formula gives results that are way off the others; it is the least accurate because it is based only on weight and does not correct for height or age. The online calculator produces numbers that are about the same as those from the Harris-Benedict equation, which is reassuring since it uses that formula. Scientists consider the Schofield results to be the most accurate, but in our case they differ from Harris-Benedict results only by about 5 percent. This means that online BMR calculators give estimates that are good enough—our favorite phrase—for most purposes.

THE UNFORTUNATE EFFECT OF AGE

The Schofield equations are more accurate because they acknowledge that the BMR varies according to age as well as sex and body size. The BMR tends to be low in early infancy, but it rises quickly during the first year of life. It declines during childhood and adolescence and remains relatively constant from about age twenty to fifty. After about age fifty or so, the great tragedy occurs: the BMR gradually declines by about 1 to 3 percent per decade. This circumstance, most likely due to age-related changes in body composition, explains why people who reach middle age find that they can no longer eat as much as they used to without putting on weight.

The BMR of women is about 6 percent lower than that of men throughout life, a difference that can be accounted for by women's higher body fat levels. When calorie requirements are related to fat-free body weight, sex differences largely disappear. Body fat is much less metabolically active than other body tissues, and its heat production accounts for only a small part of the BMR. In one study, for example, body fat accounted for nearly 14 percent of body weight but only 4 percent of the BMR. In contrast, the brain, liver, heart, and kidneys, which together constituted 6 percent of body weight, accounted for 58 percent of the BMR.[9]

The calorie cost of basal metabolism is a large—if not the largest—component of energy expenditure in all but the most active people. There is not a whole lot you or anyone else can do to increase your BMR, except by developing a higher proportion of lean to fat tissue through physical activity. Going by the results of the Schofield formula, Marion Nestle must eat about 1,200 calories a day to support her basic metabolic functions, and Malden Nesheim must eat about 1,800 to support his. These are the minimum number of calories needed to support our body functions at our particular heights, weights, ages, and stages of life. Even so, to maintain our body weights, we must eat more than these amounts. How much more depends mostly on our levels of physical activity and, to a much smaller extent, the kinds of food we eat, the matter that we take up next.

CHAPTER 7

The Second Use

Heat Losses while Metabolizing Food

One reason why basal metabolic rates must be measured when you have not eaten for twelve to fourteen hours is that eating itself raises heat production even when you are at rest. Not only that, but it usually takes several hours before your heat production returns to basal levels. You get to choose what to call this effect. In 1902 Max Rubner called it specific dynamic action (SDA). Henry Armsby called it the heat increment. More recent investigators prefer to call it the *thermic* effect of food, and we do too. These calories appear to be wasted. They are not trapped in ATP molecules and are unavailable for powering muscle activity. But they do help to keep the body warm, as you can easily notice after eating a big meal. Some investigators believe that the thermic effects of food may help to regulate body weight, an idea we return to in chapter 18.

Thermic effects arise from the acts of digesting and metabolizing food. Digestion, however, wastes very few calories. Sir Hans Krebs, who won a Nobel Prize in 1953 for his mapping of energy-producing biochemical pathways in the body (now known as the Krebs cycle), evaluated the amount of heat lost during the digestion of proteins into amino acids, fats into fatty acids, and complex carbohydrates into sugars. He demonstrated that these enzymatic actions occur readily and generate only tiny amounts of heat. By his calculations, only about 0.6 percent of the energy stored in proteins and carbohydrates is lost as heat in the digestive tract. The amount lost by fat digestion is even less, only about 0.1 percent of the original energy. These amounts are so small that they can be ignored in all but the most precise research studies.

In reviewing Krebs's studies some years later, Harold Mitchell explained, "The mastication of food, and its propulsion through the alimentary canal, the secretory activity of the digestive glands, and the absorption of the end products of digestion are types of physiological work that must result in increased heat dissipation. However, the increased heat emission is so inappreciable that it is difficult to demonstrate experimentally; or if it is demonstrated, the effect is so small . . . as to amount to an insignificant item in the total."[1]

Today it is clear that nearly all the thermic effects of food occur once the products of digestion are absorbed into the body's working area and undergo metabolism. Furthermore, the amount of heat generated during metabolism depends on which food components are being metabolized. Amino acids, fatty acids, and sugars vary in their thermic effects. Amino acids generate the most heat losses, sometimes as much as 20 to 30 percent of the calories contained in the original protein source. Fatty acids generate the least: 0 to 5 percent of the original fat calories. Sugars generate something in between; they dissipate 5 to 10 percent of the energy in the original food carbohydrates as heat.[2] The higher heat losses of amino acids seem most likely due to the energy costs of constructing urea and other molecules as a means to excrete nitrogen or of using amino acids to synthesize new body proteins.

What does this mean in dietary terms? The human diet rarely contains pure or even almost pure protein, fat, or carbohydrate. Salad oils, butter, and sugar are rare exceptions. Even in high-protein soybean curds (tofu), half the calories are from fat. Mostly, we eat foods and meals that contain highly variable mixtures of different kinds of ingredients—what nutritionists refer to as mixed diets.

Mitchell reviewed evaluations of the heat losses that occurred when people ate mixed diets containing large proportions of steak (relatively rich in protein), butter (fat), or potatoes (mostly carbohydrate). His conclusion: the thermic effects of mixed diets average out to about 10 percent of the calories available in the original foods—those that remain after accounting for losses in feces and urine.[3] The particular mix of proteins, fats, and carbohydrates does not make much of a difference to thermal losses because typical diets usually provide only 10 to 15 percent of their calories from protein.

A NEW TERM: NET METABOLIZABLE ENERGY

As we discussed in chapter 3, the Atwater Values constitute available (or metabolizable) energy—the calories available to the body *after* food is digested and absorbed and nitrogen is excreted in urine. Consequently, Atwater Values account for the indigestibility of certain components typically found in such foods as cereals, fruits, and vegetables. But in computing the number of *usable* calories in foods, it is necessary to subtract the calories wasted as heat from Atwater Values. The calories that remain are those that are available to support basal metabolism, muscle activity, and growth, pregnancy, and lactation. These constitute the net energy of the food, or as some call it, the net metabolizable energy. We illustrate the relationships among the various stages of calorie availability in figure 9.

Determining the net energy available in food requires correction for the very small heat losses of digestion (less than 1 percent) and the more substantive thermic effects of food (about 10 percent). For someone consuming a 2,000-calorie diet, the thermic effects will amount to about 200 calories. The size of this correction—and the substantial variations in the thermic effects of consuming proteins, fats, and carbohydrates—induced the British food scientist Geoffrey Livesey to challenge the continued use of Atwater Values.

Livesey minces no words. The theoretical basis of the Atwater Values, he says, is "totally flawed," "anachronistic," and at best "an approximate surrogate of available energy." He insists that the measurement of calories in food must account not only for the indigestibility of food carbohydrates and their fermentation by intestinal bacteria but also for differences in the amounts of heat lost by the specific food components.[4]

To account for these sources of error, Livesey proposes replacing Atwater's available (or metabolizable) energy with the more precise net metabolizable energy, based on his own calculations of the thermic effects of food. Table 8 gives Livesey's proposed factors. By *available carbohydrate* he means complex carbohydrates (starches) and sugars. By *fermentable carbohydrate* he means dietary fiber and certain "resistant" starches that are impervious to human digestive enzymes but can be digested by the enzymatic action of intestinal bacteria.

Livesey's values for available carbohydrate and fat are close to the Atwater Values for those components. The calorie values of protein, however, are quite

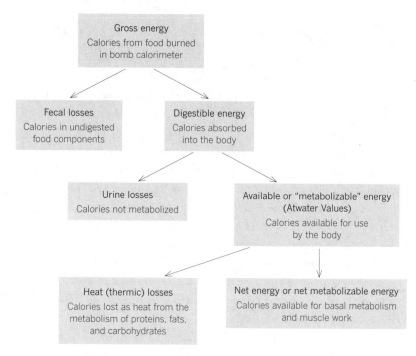

FIGURE 9. Net energy, or net metabolizable energy, corrects for heat losses that occur during metabolism—the thermic effects of food.

different in Atwater's and Livesey's approaches. The net metabolizable energy values for protein-rich foods are lower in Livesey's calculations because of the higher heat loss of protein in metabolism. But as we just explained, the metabolic heat losses for mixed diets—which are what people actually eat—tend to average out to about 10 percent of the original calories (because protein usually accounts for only a small fraction of total calorie intake). How important is a 10 percent difference? Because errors in estimating the calories in foods and in daily diets are often much greater than 10 percent, it constitutes a relatively small error by comparison. For this reason, we are not convinced that Livesey's figures for individual food components matter very much for ordinary people consuming ordinary diets.

Although Livesey believes that national and international agencies should use his values rather than Atwater's, he has been unable to persuade them to do so. In 2002 the United Nations' Food and Agriculture Organization (FAO) called a meeting of international experts, including Livesey, to con-

TABLE 8   COMPARISON OF LIVESEY'S NET
METABOLIZABLE ENERGY TO ATWATER VALUES
(METABOLIZABLE ENERGY), CALORIES PER GRAM

Component	Livesey's net metabolizable energy	Atwater Values (metabolizable energy)
Protein	3.2	4
Fat	8.9	9
Available carbohydrate	3.8	4
Fermentable carbohydrate	1.9	4

sider whether the replacement of Atwater Values with net metabolizable energy would be feasible and, if so, useful. The group produced a long and highly detailed report with which Livesey apparently concurred. Here is our blunt summary of the report's conclusions: changing to Livesey's values is possible, but why bother?

The report points out that estimates of daily energy requirements throughout the world are based on the Atwater Values. To change the values at this point would be painful to accomplish. Atwater Values have been used to calculate the content of infant formulas, the information given in food composition tables, the results of dietary intake surveys, and historical surveys of food and nutrient availability. They are the basis of calories listed on food labels in the United States. All would need to be recalculated. Consumers who have gotten accustomed to using the Atwater Values of 4, 9, and 4 calories per gram for proteins, fats, and carbohydrates would need to be reeducated—and would be required to learn new numbers that use decimal points, no less. And because the switch would have to take place in all of these areas at exactly the same time, it would be a great burden not only to government staff but also to the food industry.

Yes, fixing this situation would be annoying, but wouldn't it be worth the trouble to have more accurate values? The expert committee considered this question and concluded that there was little justification for making the switch. It was not only the high potential cost of the change that bothered the committee members. They were much more convinced by the trivial size of the benefit. As the report explained, "In most cases the error incurred will be about 5 percent, which is within the usually accepted limits of measurement error or biological variation."[5] Our translation: Atwater Values are good enough for most practical—if not research—purposes. The size of the errors in Atwater Values hardly matters when compared to the much larger errors involved in estimating the nutrient content of food or the number of calories people consume and use each day.

The expert committee did not entirely reject the idea of dropping the Atwater Values and replacing them with net metabolizable energy. It just postponed that discussion for a later time: "There was uniform agreement, however, that the issue should continue to be discussed in the future, and that it could profitably be revisited during workshops and expert consultations involving recommendations, assessment of adequacy, public health policy, etc. surrounding food and dietary energy. This would assure that scientists in a variety of disciplines, regulators, and policy-makers have an opportunity to explore more thoroughly the merits and implications of making such a change when it is deemed appropriate."[6]

REGULATING BODY TEMPERATURE

Some of the heat produced by the metabolism of food and by metabolism in general is used to regulate body temperature. More energy is needed for this purpose when the ambient temperatures are hot enough to induce sweating or cold enough to induce shivering. But in modern societies, people usually adjust their clothing to compensate for extreme temperatures or keep their surroundings heated or air-conditioned. Under ordinary circumstances, additional energy is not needed to maintain body temperatures. Or, to put it the way we usually do, not enough additional energy is needed to make much overall difference in calculating energy needs.

To repeat: the thermic effects of food—on the order of 10 percent—are small relative to the energy cost of basal metabolism, which usually accounts for about two-thirds of daily caloric needs. The other third or so—or, sometimes, much more—derives from the energy costs of physical activity, the matter to which we now turn.

CHAPTER 8

The Third Use
Physical Activity

Physical activities—the normal moving around that you do during daily life and the more intense actions involved in deliberate exercise—promote good health. Using calories to be active is well established to strengthen muscles, help maintain body weight within healthy ranges, reduce risk factors for chronic disease, and make you feel better.

The amount of physical activity most closely associated with these benefits is a matter of some debate, but most authorities advise you to regularly engage in moderate or vigorous activity for at least half an hour on most days.[1] By *moderate activity*, they mean the equivalent of brisk walking. By *vigorous*, they mean jogging or its equivalent. This amount is more, sometimes much more, than most people do. Even so, the calories required to power this level of recommended activity are likely to add up to only a small percentage of those required for basal metabolism. Their number is also small relative to the calories that most people eat in a day.

This, however, does not stop food companies and government agencies from emphasizing physical activity as the primary strategy for maintaining or losing body weight. From a political standpoint, advice to move more is much less threatening than advice to eat less. Moving more does not affect the economic interests of food companies or any other powerful industry. In contrast, as we keep reminding you, eating less is bad for business. And advice to eat less raises uncomfortable questions about exactly what foods you are supposed to eat less of. With that said, we must make it clear that we think it is important to be as physically active as possible, but mainly for health reasons that go beyond just balancing food calories.

In the previous two chapters we counted the calories required to maintain basal metabolism and to metabolize food. These amounts can be measured or estimated with reasonable precision. Scientists, for example, can estimate basal metabolic requirements using fairly decent formulas that consider body size, age, and sex. They can assume that no more than 10 percent of the calories in food are wasted as heat and can ignore the small amount of additional energy that might be needed to maintain body temperature in extreme heat or cold. For most people these calories add up to about two-thirds of the total number needed to be consumed each day to maintain a healthy body weight. The remaining "third" is needed to compensate for spontaneous or intentional physical activity. "Third" goes in quotation marks because people vary greatly in their activity levels and activity levels vary substantially from day to day. Among people who are extremely active, the energy expended in physical activity can exceed basal energy expenditures by a factor of two or more.

ATWATER'S EARLY ESTIMATIONS

In 1894 Wilbur Atwater and his colleagues published summaries of studies conducted by his group but also by investigators throughout the world who were trying to define dietary standards for men of various occupations. By *dietary standards*, Atwater meant the number of calories required to support a person's daily needs. These studies were based on records of dietary intake. Investigators of his era and earlier observed that most people maintained a relatively constant body weight over time. As a result, they could assume that calorie intake was an accurate estimation of calorie expenditure and requirements. Indeed it can be, but *only* among people whose weight does not vary over time. Table 9 gives some examples of Atwater's observations.[2]

The number of calories recorded as consumed—and, therefore, assumed to be expended—ranged from the 2,200 per day required by underfed laborers in Italy to the 5,600 reported by hard-working machinists. On average, men performing light activity required 3,000 calories a day, whereas those engaged in heavy activity required more than 4,000. Despite the use of dietary records to determine calorie expenditure and the difficulty of obtaining international publications in those ancient, pre-Internet days, Atwater's

TABLE 9   ATWATER'S "DIETARY STANDARDS" FOR MEN
AT VARYING LEVELS OF ACTIVITY

Level of activity	Calories per day
Individuals	
Underfed laborers, Italy	2,200
College students, U.S.	2,600
Mechanics at moderate work, Sweden	3,000
Laborers at active work, England	3,600
Miners at severe work, Prussia	3,800
Mechanics at severe work, Sweden	4,200
Machinists at hard work, Connecticut	5,600
Averages	
Man with light exercise	2,980
Man with moderate muscular work	3,520
Man with active muscular work	4,060

SOURCE: Atwater and Langworthy, 1897 (see note 2).

1894 conclusions about calorie needs are quite close to the more precise figures obtained in recent years from doubly labeled water measurements (as we explain in the next chapter).

THE INTENSITY EFFECT

Even in the 1890s, Atwater was able to show that the number of calories used in physical activity depended on the intensity of effort as well as on body weight. These days, exercise physiologists can measure the number of calories expended in a wide range of physical activities using portable oxygen uptake devices. Because larger bodies need more calories to support basal metabolic needs as well as physical activities, physiologists must correct oxygen uptake measurements for body weight.[3] The more recent and more accurate studies of the energy expended by men and women of various sizes and shapes confirm Atwater's observations. They show that at any body weight, the energy cost of an activity depends on its intensity. This is intuitively obvious. It takes more energy to walk up stairs than it does to walk on a flat surface. The more effort put into an activity, the more calories it requires. Table 10 shows the effect of intensity.

TABLE 10   CALORIES USED IN DAILY ACTIVITIES OF
VARYING INTENSITY

Activity	Calories per minute*	Level of exertion
Activities of daily living		
Lying down; riding in a vehicle	1.0	Sedentary
Watering plants	2.5	Mild
Taking out trash; walking dog	3.0	Moderate
Raking lawn	4.0	Moderate
Gardening (no lifting)	4.4	Moderate
Chopping wood	4.9	Vigorous
Walking at various rates		
Walking 2 mph	2.5	Mild
Walking 3 mph	3.3	Moderate
Walking 4 mph	4.5	Moderate
Walking 5 mph	8.0	Vigorous

SOURCE: Adapted from IOM, 2005: table 1-12 (see note 3).

*These figures are specific to a person who weighs 57 kilograms (125 pounds). Expenditures are lower for people who weigh less and higher for those who weigh more.

To put the figures in this table in perspective, suppose you are a 125-pound woman and you consume one 12-ounce soft drink in excess of your daily calorie needs. To balance the 150 calories it contains through the level of activity involved in walking, you would need to walk for:

- ✦ 60 minutes at 2 miles per hour (and, obviously, cover 2 miles)
- ✦ 45 minutes at 3 miles per hour (and cover more than 2 miles)
- ✦ 19 minutes at 5 miles per hour (and cover 1.5 miles)

Another example: if you are lucky enough to live in one of the dozens of cities served by the transit direction Website HopStop.com, you can type in where you are and where you plan to go and find out how many calories it will cost you to walk there. Marion Nestle used the site to count calories from her Manhattan home to the nearest farmers' market, 0.53 mile away—a mere 41 calories. Although this figure is not adjusted for body weight or intensity, it confirms our point: balancing calorie intake with physical activity takes considerable effort. Unfortunately, overeating calories takes hardly any effort at all. That is the principal reason why calorie intake dominates expenditure as the more critical factor in weight loss.

TABLE II   INCREASE IN ENERGY EXPENDITURE WITH
INCREASING INTENSITY AND BODY WEIGHT

Running intensity		Body weight, pounds		
		130	155	190
Miles per hour	Minutes per mile	Calories per minute*		
5	12.0	8	10	12
6	10.0	10	11	14
7	8.5	11	13	16
8	7.5	12	14	17
9	6.5	13	15	18
10	6.0	15	17	21
11	5.5	16	19	23

SOURCE: Calculated from Ainsworth et al., 2011 (see note 4). The figures are acceptable for survey research but do not consider individual variations in body fat, age, sex, efficiency of movement, or geographic and environmental conditions that might affect energy expenditure.

*Figures rounded off to nearest calorie.

THE EFFECT OF BODY WEIGHT

The one advantage of being overweight is that you expend more calories in physical movement. Larger bodies take more energy to move. The energy cost of running illustrates the effect of body weight on calorie expenditure, as shown in table II.[4]

Suppose you are a 130-pound woman running a 10-minute mile. If so, you will expend 10 calories for every minute you run, or 600 calories per hour. At any speed, you will be using about 100 calories per mile. In contrast, if you are a 190-pound man, you will be burning 14 calories per minute and 840 in an hour. At any speed, you will be expending about 150 calories per mile. And if you are a 155-pound marathoner running 5.5-minute miles, you will expend just under 3,000 calories in the 2.5 hours you are on the road. This is almost enough to burn off a pound of fat, which is either a little or a lot depending on how you look at it. At the lower end of running intensity, the number of calories required is much, much less. As important as physical activity is for health, you have to do a lot of it, and intensely, to compensate for excessive calorie intake.

At the far extreme of intensity, physical activity can more than compensate for overeating. The most intense physical activity recorded over limited periods of time is observed in bicyclists competing in the Tour de France. These elite cyclists are estimated to expend an astonishing 8,100 calories per day for the 21 days of the race. Men hauling sleds across the Arctic have been found to expend about 7,900 calories per day over a 20-day period. Sustainable energy expenditures of a more imaginable 4,000 calories per day have been measured among individuals in such diverse groups as soldiers in training, lumberjacks, and coal miners.[5] As long as people keep up this level of activity, their problem will be maintaining weight, not gaining it.

THE "EXTRA ENERGY FROM PHYSICAL ACTIVITY"

The calorie cost of engaging in physical activities does not completely account for the full calorie benefit of intentional exercise or intense work. For some hours—perhaps as many as fifteen—following intense physical exertion, calorie expenditure continues to exceed basal levels. This is one of the reasons why measurements of basal metabolism must be taken at rest and many hours after physical activity. Physiologists have a name for this increased calorie expenditure: excess post-exercise oxygen consumption (EPOC).[6] As you might expect, the EPOC depends on the intensity and the duration of the activity. It also depends on body weight.

At most, the extra EPOC energy accounts for an additional 15 percent of calories expended in the activity itself. For long-distance power walkers or runners, this would raise the number of calories used per mile to 115 for a lighter person and 170 for a heavier person. While we like to use 100 calories per mile as a ballpark figure to explain the energy cost of physical activity, this number is too high for the average sedentary person. If you are a slow walker, you probably do not expend more than half a calorie per pound of body weight per mile. If you weigh 150 pounds, the energy you use while strolling along will be just 75 calories per mile.

THE ENERGY COST OF FIDGETING

What physiologists prefer to call spontaneous non-exercise activity—fidgeting—has been found to account for an impressive 100 to 800 calories a day. These figures are not just estimated. They have been measured in people confined in whole-body calorimeters. Some people are just more fidgety than

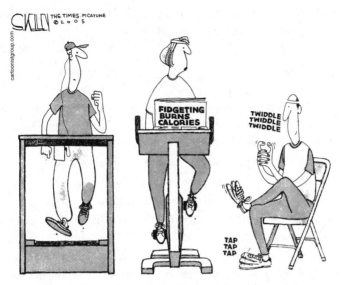

FIGURE 10. Some people seem to be able to eat a lot without gaining weight. Spontaneous non-exercise activity, also known as fidgeting, may explain this phenomenon. © Steve Kelley, used with permission of Steve Kelley and Creators Syndicate. All rights reserved.

others and use up more calories that way. Fidgeting may well explain why your best friend can eat enormous meals and stay lean while you seem to put on weight if you even think about eating, as illustrated in figure 10.

Scientists who research such things observe that infants who were overweight by the time they reached their first birthday had been expending 21 percent less energy during that first year than their normal-weight counterparts. Because the researchers did not observe any innate differences in basal metabolic rates among the infants, they attributed the differences in body weights to lower levels of spontaneous physical activity. Studies like this suggest that the degree of fidgeting has some genetic basis and might well be related to the propensity for weight gain and obesity throughout life.[7]

Additional evidence supports this idea. Investigators in Cambridge, England, studied infants born to overweight mothers. They took measurements of energy expenditure when the babies were three months old and again when the babies had reached one year of age. Infants in the lowest 20 percent of calorie expenditure were much more likely to be overweight by their first birthday, even though their calorie intake was about the same as that of leaner infants. But evidence in adults argues that total calorie intake is by far the dominant determinant of weight gain.[8]

THE ENERGY COST OF MENTAL EFFORT

We thought we should end this chapter with a comment about the amount of energy you are using to read this book. The brain has high requirements for energy. On average, the heat produced by the brain accounts for fully 20 percent of the energy expended in basal metabolism. The brain uses the energy metabolized from 150 to 200 grams of glucose every day—400 to 600 calories. But if you just want to sit around and think about physical activity, you will not be using many additional calories. This too has been investigated, and long ago.

In the early 1900s Francis Benedict concluded from his calorimeter studies of human volunteers that mental effort has little effect on the brain's energy use or on energy use in general. When he measured the energy expended by his study subjects at rest or engaged in sustained mental effort (solving difficult multiplication problems, for example), he could account for most of the increase in heat they were producing by the effects of their more rapid heartbeats and more tightly clenched muscles. T. L. Sourkes found that solving simple mathematical problems increased heat production over basal levels by fewer than 8 calories per hour. Solving more complicated problems for an hour doubled that number, to the equivalent of the calories in one teaspoon of sugar.[9] Malden Nesheim attended a class led by the twentieth-century nutritionist H. H. Mitchell in which he assured the students that they could easily accomplish an hour of mental work on the calories produced by half a peanut.

With the energy costs of physical—and mental—activity well in hand, let's move on to part 3 and add up the number of calories you might need each day to balance the total cost of basal metabolism, the thermic effect of food, and additional physical activity.

PART THREE

Calorie Intake and Its Regulation

It is now time to consider questions about the number of calories really needed in the course of everyday life, the number people are actually consuming, and the ways in which the body controls calorie intake. Because scientists know a great deal about the energy requirements of basal metabolism and physical activities, they have been able to develop equations that give reasonably accurate estimates of the basal metabolic rate and the total energy expenditures of men and women of differing weights, heights, ages, and physical activity levels. These equations have proved to be useful for estimating energy needs under a variety of conditions, especially because actual measurements of calorie requirements can only be done with equipment or techniques that are complicated, inconvenient, and expensive.

Wilbur Atwater devoted considerable thought to how he might estimate the calorie needs of individuals when their diets and activities varied so much from day to day, as did their ways of handling what they ate. In the 1894 *Yearbook* of the Department of Agriculture he wrote:

> Just why individuals differ in their ways of utilizing their food, and how to measure the differences and make dietary rules to fit them exactly, are problems which the physiological chemist of today is far from solving. The fact is that the whole subject is new, and the accurate investigation thus far made, though quite considerable when we get it all together, is far too small for satisfactory conclusions. The best we can do with our present knowledge, or rather lack of knowledge, of the subject is to make general estimates, with the clear understanding that they are only rough estimates, and that they apply to average rather than individual cases. (p. 369)

Much has improved since Atwater's time. Nevertheless, equations are still just estimates. In a real sense, they are guesses. How close the guesses come to measured values is a matter of much conjecture, but they can be off by double-digit percentages. In dealing with calorie estimates, we think it helps to become comfortable with rather large degrees of uncertainty. The idea that an uncertainty in calorie estimates of 10 percent or more can be ignored is enough to induce discomfort, if not dismay, in many people. You might, for example, view as ridiculous the idea that everyone continues to use the Atwater Values despite their demonstrable imprecision.

We agree that it would be easier to talk about calories if they could be discussed more precisely. And as the chapters in this section should make clear, precise measurements of calorie intake and expenditure are possible when done carefully in laboratory studies. But short of calorimeter and doubly labeled water investigations, talking about calories means talking about estimates. From our reading of the research, it seems clear that some estimates are better than others, but overall we have come to believe that most estimates are good enough for most practical purposes.

In this part of the book we discuss how physiologists estimate the calorie requirements of men and women who vary in age, size, shape, food intake, and activity level. We explain why it is so difficult to find out what people eat—as opposed to what they *say* they eat. And we at last get to the number of calories provided by alcoholic beverages. Finally, we take up the matter of how calorie intake is regulated so that your body knows when you have eaten enough to meet your requirements. If there is a theme to this discussion, it is surely that the human body does a superb job of making sure that it gets enough calories to meet biological needs but is much less effective at knowing when calories are in excess. The result is that it is much easier for you and everyone else to overeat than to stop eating when you are no longer hungry.

CHAPTER 9

How Many Calories Do You Need?

We can't think of any intuitive way to answer this question. When everything is working the way it should, you don't need to give calorie requirements a thought. You eat when you are hungry, you stop when you are full, your weight does not change, and somehow it all works out. About all you can do to sense calories is feel full after eating and realize that it takes more energy to work up a sweat than to sit at a desk.

As to the number of calories you need, they must balance the number you expend. A United Nations expert group puts this more formally: "The energy requirement of an individual is the level of energy intake from food that will balance energy expenditure when the individual has a body size and composition, and level of physical activity, consistent with long-term good health; and that will allow for the maintenance of economically necessary and socially desirable physical activity. In children and pregnant or lactating women the energy requirement includes the energy needs associated with the deposition of tissues or the secretion of milk at rates consistent with good health."[1]

We particularly like "economically necessary and socially desirable physical activity," but overall we view this and all other such definitions as tautologies: you need as much energy as you need. If you are not gaining or losing weight, the number of calories you eat over time should be the same as the number you expend. To estimate total calorie requirements, physiologists and nutrition researchers separately estimate and add together each component of energy expenditure—the basal metabolic rate (BMR), the heat

TABLE 12   AVERAGE BASAL AND TOTAL ENERGY
EXPENDITURES FOR MALES AND FEMALES, BY AGE

Age in years	Basal metabolic rate (BMR)	Total energy expenditure (TEE)
Males		
3–8	1,040	1,440
9–13	1,320	2,080
14–18	1,730	3,120
19–30	1,770	3,080
31–50	1,680	3,020
51–70	1,530	2,470
71+	1,480	2,240
Females		
3–8	1,010	1,490
9–13	1,190	1,910
14–18	1,360	2,300
19–30	1,360	2,440
31–50	1,320	2,410
51–70	1,230	2,070
71+	1,190	1,570

SOURCE: Adapted from IOM, 2005: table 5-10 (see note 3).
NOTE: Expenditures rounded off to the nearest 10 calories. These figures are specific to moderately active people whose weights are within normal ranges. Adults age 19 and over: BMRs are measured values, and TEEs were measured using doubly labeled water. Children: Figures were calculated from equations based on age, height, and weight.

effects of food, the energy expended in physical activity, and the additional increments due to fidgeting or to longer-term effects of activity. This should and often does give a number that comes close to calorimeter measurements.

Since Wilbur Atwater's era, scientists have been able to measure—as opposed to estimate—total energy output using whole-body calorimeters or portable oxygen consumption devices. In recent years they have increasingly used doubly labeled water to measure energy use in study subjects going about their normal daily activities for periods of two to three weeks. Researchers have now collected the results of doubly labeled water experiments done on hundreds of men and women of various ages. In table 12, we summarize the average values found in doubly labeled water studies of one specific category of people: those who are moderately active and whose weights fall within ranges considered normal.[2]

Take a look at the figures that might best apply to you. The table illustrates several key points:

- At every age, men have higher basal and total energy expenditures than women.
- Adult men expend an average of about 3,050 calories per day; adult women expend about 2,400 calories per day (if moderately active and neither underweight nor overweight).
- Basal and total energy expenditures increase throughout childhood, reach a peak from ages 14 to 30, and then decline with increasing age.
- Basal metabolism accounts for 50 to 70 percent of total energy expenditure throughout life.
- Even by age 9, the total energy expenditure of boys and girls is close to 2,000 calories per day.

We must emphasize that the numbers of calories in this table are *measured* values obtained in research studies. Such studies are complicated to manage and can only be done with limited numbers of volunteers. Nevertheless, the results are instructive. For example, table 12 indicates that from age 14 to 50, the measured energy expenditures of men and women exceed amounts reported in dietary intake surveys by several hundred calories a day. Measured expenditures also substantially exceed the FDA's 2,000-calorie-a-day standard, a level used on food labels and for calorie postings on restaurant menus (see chapter 23).

ESTIMATED ENERGY REQUIREMENT (EER)

Nutrition scientists can measure the BMR and calories expended in physical activity, add them up, and calculate the total energy expended by individuals. But this number does not necessarily reflect the number of calories required to maintain an appropriate body weight. Nutritionists do not define precise standards for appropriate levels of calorie intake. We can't. People vary too much in dietary intake and physical activity levels to set meaningful levels. Instead, we use something called the estimated energy requirement (EER). This we define as the average daily intake of calories needed to maintain a healthy and relatively constant body weight in men and women of various ages, weights, heights, physical activity levels, and life stages. Vague enough? The EER is a frank admission that estimating calorie requirements is a

TABLE 13   ESTIMATED ENERGY EXPENDITURES OF
MEN AND WOMEN OF VARYING BODY WEIGHTS AND
ACTIVITY LEVELS, CALORIES PER DAY

	Sedentary	Very active
Male, 5'11", 30 years old		
154 pounds	2,510	3,530
250 pounds	3,090	4,450
Female, 5'5", 30 years old		
129 pounds	1,900	2,680
210 pounds	2,300	3,260

SOURCE: Adapted from IOM, 2005: tables 5-29 and 5-30 (see note 3).
NOTE: Calories rounded to the nearest 10.

chancy business. It depends on physical activity levels, which are of course highly variable, but also on more stable factors that also vary, such as:

+ *Age:* Energy expenditure declines from peak levels with age, by as much as 20 percent by age 50 and 30 percent by age 71+. Although basal metabolic rates also decline with age, most of the drop comes from reduced physical activity. Whether an increase in physical activity can fully compensate for the decline is uncertain. It seems to help but may not be enough.

+ *Body composition:* Lean muscle tissue uses more calories for its weight than does fatty tissue. Among people with equivalent body weights, those with the higher fat mass will expend fewer calories, since body fat is much less metabolically active than muscle or other lean tissues.

+ *Sex:* Women use fewer calories for their body weights than do men. This is primarily due to the higher proportion of body fat in women but may also be due to differences in hormonal status.

+ *Weight status:* Doubly labeled water experiments show that both the BMR and the total energy expenditure (including physical activity) *increase* with increasing overweight or obesity. Despite the relatively lower energy cost of maintaining body fat, heavier bodies take more energy to maintain and to move. The increase in basal and total expenditure with weight appears to hold true at any level of physical activity. The effect of weight can amount to hundreds of calories a day, as shown in table 13.

Face it. The EER is imprecise and can never be a biological constant. If your body weight stays pretty much the same, your estimated requirement should come close to the average total energy expenditure for someone of your sex and age. For most people, the average estimates will vary from actual requirements but are probably within an acceptable range of error. Using these figures is a lot easier than signing up for calorimeter or doubly labeled water experiments, more accurate as they may be. The one factor that might make a significant difference is if your life stage involves growth, pregnancy, or lactation.

THE INCREASED ENERGY NEEDS OF GROWTH, PREGNANCY, AND LACTATION

Anyone who has ever lived with an adolescent boy might imagine that his increased calorie needs must be enormous. You might also think that the energy cost of producing an infant or breast milk must be equally massive. When measured, however, the increments in energy needs turn out to be small relative to the large energy costs of basal metabolism and physical activity. For example, scientists estimate that the average increase in energy needed to support the growth of children is just 20 calories a day, rising to 30 calories a day or so during periods of peak growth.[3] The voracious appetites of adolescent boys are better explained by their higher BMRs and higher expenditures in physical activity than by the calorie needs of growth.

In the case of pregnancy, the proverbial "eating for two" is not quite right. The energy needs of the fetus are small relative to the mother's basal energy requirements and activity costs, especially during the first trimester. Energy needs rise during later stages of pregnancy. The BMR rises because of the additional metabolic needs of the fetus itself and of the mother's uterus, the placenta, and the extra work performed by the heart, lungs, and kidneys to deal with her expanded blood volume. The weight gain that accompanies pregnancy also causes the expenditure of more energy during physical activity.

The Institute of Medicine's summary of this situation suggests that the energy needs of pregnant women do not change much in the first trimester. By the second trimester, however, they supposedly increase by about 340 calories per day, and then by 450 calories a day in the third trimester. These are substantial and generous increases that should more than account for the calorie needs of the fetus and its surrounding tissues as well as the additional pounds that most women put on during pregnancy. For many women, such increments are higher than necessary and will promote excessive weight gain.

The energy requirement of lactation depends on the volume of milk produced. During the first six months of breastfeeding, an additional 500 calories a day covers the energy needs of milk production. But according to the Institute of Medicine and other experts, about 170 of those calories are drawn from the mother's fat reserves, meaning that she only needs to eat an additional 330 calories a day beyond her usual energy requirements. After about six months of breastfeeding, the mother's need for additional energy drops to about 400 calories a day, increasingly derived from the diet.[4] As always, these are average values that vary with individual weights, activity levels, and other such factors.

THE FDA'S 2,000-CALORIE STANDARD

Food package labels and restaurant menus in the United States use diets of 2,000 calories a day as the basis for evaluating intake of foods and meals. As we explain in more detail in chapter 23, the FDA originally intended to use 2,350 calories as the basis for comparison when it wrote the regulations for Nutrition Facts labels in 1993. This reflected the average number of calories reported as consumed in the USDA's dietary intake surveys of the time. But those who commented on the FDA's proposal did not like this number. They predicted that a 2,350-calorie standard would encourage overeating, especially among women. Instead, they suggested 2,000 as easier to use, consistent with popular food plans, and closer to the energy needs of postmenopausal women, a key target group for obesity prevention. They argued that the lower number would be more likely to help consumers understand that they might need more or less than 2,000 calories a day and should choose foods according to their own dietary needs.

As an alternative, some advisors to the FDA suggested that the agency list calories in ranges similar to those reported in the USDA's dietary intake surveys. Food labels, they said, should include a statement that "typical intakes for women are 1,600 to 2,200 calories, for men 2,000 to 3,000 calories, and for children (ages 4 to 14), 1,800 to 2,500 calories." Note that these figures are somewhat lower than the estimates for daily calorie needs given in table 13. In any case, the FDA rejected the range idea. It did not view ranges as less likely to confuse or mislead the public. Instead, the FDA selected the 2,000-calorie standard and dealt with the range issue by listing diets of 2,000 and 2,500 calories on package labels.[5]

By now it should be evident that 2,000 calories is much lower than either measurements or estimates of the total energy needs of all but the smallest and most sedentary people. We did warn you that these kinds of imprecisions might make you uncomfortable. Without participating in calorimeter, oxygen consumption, or doubly labeled water experiments, the best you can do is try to do better in estimating your total calorie needs. But surely it ought to be possible to measure the number of calories you eat? And shouldn't your calorie intake indicate the number you need? We consider those questions next.

CHAPTER 10

Calorie Confusion

The Struggle to Estimate Intake

As we demonstrated in the previous chapter, studies using doubly labeled water—as close to a gold standard as exists—find that the average non-overweight adult man needs about 3,050 calories a day to maintain a stable body weight, and the average woman about 2,400. The FDA's 2,000-calorie standard for food labels is 50 percent lower than the average for men and 20 percent lower than that for women. But many—if not most—Americans are gaining weight. Therefore, they must be eating more calories each day than they need to maintain a stable weight. (How many more? See chapter 17.)

Research on diet and health in general, and on weight gain in particular, depends on knowing what people eat. But outside of a whole-body calorimeter or a controlled environment for metabolic studies, getting even reasonably accurate information about dietary intake is, to say the least, challenging. Indeed, we consider finding out what people eat the greatest intellectual challenge in the field of nutrition today. Why? We have no nice way of saying this. Whether consciously or unconsciously, most people cannot or do not give accurate information about what they eat. When it comes to dietary intake, pretty much everyone forgets or dissembles. This problem makes surveys of dietary intake exceedingly difficult to conduct and to interpret.

DIETARY INTAKE SURVEYS

As we keep saying, doubly labeled water methods make it possible—although at considerable effort and expense—to measure average calorie expenditures in individuals going about their daily lives for periods of up to about three weeks. The number of people whose calorie needs can be determined this way is limited. To date, scientists have not come up with any simple, inexpensive way to measure calorie intake accurately in large groups of individuals who are not incarcerated in a laboratory but are "free-living" and going about the normal business of daily life.

Short of duplicate meal analysis, a method in which chemists analyze the nutrient composition of an exact duplicate of everything someone eats, all other methods for obtaining information about dietary intake depend on self-reports. These are, again to understate the matter, inconsistent and unreliable. Merely asking people about what they eat influences what they tell investigators. Even duplicate meal analysis has its hazards, as knowing your meals will be checked can be enough to change your normal eating behavior.

The usual methods for obtaining information about dietary intake ask you to do one of three things:

+ Report what you remember eating and drinking in the previous day (this is called a retrospective twenty-four-hour diet recall).

+ Keep a record of what you eat for a day or more (concurrent diet record).

+ Mark off on a long list of foods the ones you ate within the past day, week, month, or year (retrospective food frequency questionnaire).

The lack of precision in these methods is legendary. People do not easily remember what they ate. You might forget or be uncomfortable about reporting late-night snacks, candy picked up on the run, something you ate in a car, alcoholic beverages, or the amounts of foods you are eating. Like most people, you probably tend to underestimate the sizes of your food portions and overlook intake of foods you perceive as unhealthy. And, of course, you do not eat the same foods every day.

Nutrition scientists have put enormous effort into trying to evaluate the magnitude of reporting errors. They find that people underestimate their true calorie intake by astonishing percentages, typically 30 percent, with a range of 10 to 45 percent depending on such factors as age, sex, body composition, and socioeconomic status. Underreporting of food—and therefore calorie—intake increases with age and is greater among women, people who are overweight, and those of low education and income status. People also tend to exaggerate intake of foods they think are supposed to be good for health.[1]

Researchers are still debating whether one survey method is better than another, whether collecting information about portion sizes is either useful or necessary in dietary intake surveys of populations, and indeed whether any method can capture the complexities of diets that vary so much from person to person and from day to day. As an example of how hard it is to draw conclusions from surveys based on one day's reported food intake, a decades-old study done by the USDA deserves careful attention.

THE USDA'S BELTSVILLE STUDY

The USDA runs an agricultural research center in Beltsville, Maryland. In the early 1980s its scientists observed glaring inconsistencies in the results of the agency's national surveys of dietary intake. They noticed that the number of calories reported as consumed by men and women in 1977–78 was lower than the number reported in 1965. Not only that, but respondents to the 1977–78 survey reported intakes 300 to 400 calories below the amounts needed to maintain their weights. Even more suspicious, during the thirteen-year period from 1965 to 1978 the average heights and weights of survey participants had increased, meaning that they should have been eating more calories, not fewer. USDA scientists guessed that survey participants were underreporting calorie intake and decided to study whether twenty-four-hour or even three-day dietary intake records could truly approximate habitual food intakes.

The investigators asked their fellow employees at Beltsville to volunteer for a demanding experiment: reporting everything they ate or drank every single day for one entire year. Amazingly, they were able to induce twenty-nine USDA employees working in staff, scientific, and administrative positions to sign up for this undertaking. The investigators knew that the act of reporting might influence what the volunteers ate or said they ate. As a reliability check, they also collected duplicate meals from each volunteer for one full week on four occasions during that year. They reported the results of this herculean effort in a supplement to the *American Journal of Clinical Nutrition* in 1984.[2]

The study population included thirteen men and sixteen women, ages twenty to fifty-three. They were instructed to eat as they always did but to measure the sizes and weights of everything they consumed with rulers, measuring cups, measuring spoons, and a food scale. They were also to write down brand names, food preparation methods, and recipes. From this mountain of data, the USDA scientists converted information about food intake into nutrient and calorie intake through the use of food composition tables.

The results? The men in the study reported consuming an average of 2,760 calories and the women 1,850 calories a day. Their weights did not change during the year. These figures were 200 to 300 calories higher than averages reported in dietary intake surveys of that era. Even so, the investigators knew that the calories had to be underreported. They had the proof. During the four weeks in which they analyzed duplicate meals, they found actual calories to exceed reported calories by an average of 13 percent. On this basis, they urged readers to be cautious when interpreting balance studies done with subjects consuming self-selected diets.[3]

In subsequent studies, USDA statisticians had some fun with these data. They calculated the number of days on which dietary intake data would have to be collected to arrive at an estimate of calorie intake that fell within plus or minus 10 percent of the average for the 365 days of the study. The minimum number of days? *Fourteen.* And this was for the volunteers whose diets varied least from day to day. For the group as a whole, the number of reporting days required to get within 10 percent of the average number of calories consumed was *twenty-seven.* For the man whose diet varied the most, it took *eighty-four* days of food records to get within 10 percent of his average daily calorie intake for the year.[4]

The moral: one twenty-four-hour dietary analysis is unlikely to represent average dietary intake. Given this problem, we can understand why even the most carefully conducted dietary surveys find average calorie intakes to be well below those observed in doubly labeled water studies. But researchers hope that the results of taking twenty-four-hour recalls or collecting food frequency records from large numbers of people—the more the better—will average out and indicate intake levels or dietary patterns that apply to the group as a whole, if not to specific individuals within the group.[5]

WHAT WE EAT IN AMERICA

This brings us to the large-scale surveys, published under the title *What We Eat in America,* conducted jointly by the Centers for Disease Control and Prevention (CDC) and the USDA. The CDC conducts surveys of nationally representative samples of about 8,500 people at regular intervals, and the USDA analyzes the results. The people go to a mobile examination center to be interviewed extensively—with much cross-questioning of the information they give—about what they ate during the past twenty-four hours. A second such interview, also with as much cross-checking as possible, is done by telephone.[6]

The 2008 survey reported a combined average intake for men and women of 2,070 calories a day, close to the FDA's rounded-down 2,000-calorie-per-day benchmark. Adult men (age 20 or over) were found to consume an average of about 2,500 calories a day. Adult women consumed about 1,800. These totals are 500–600 calories lower than those obtained in doubly labeled water experiments and are consistent with typical self-reporting deficits of 20 percent to 30 percent.[7] One problem with errors this large is that there is no easy way to tell whether survey participants underestimate all foods equally or single out some foods for greater underestimation. Hence: difficulties in interpretation.

CALORIES IN THE FOOD SUPPLY

A second source of information about dietary intake is indirect: data on the availability of commodities in the food supply. Food supply data are not based on what people actually eat but are instead based on the amounts of food *available* for consumption—the foods produced annually in the United States plus imports, less exports. The USDA divides these totals by the population count on a particular midyear date and presents the data as amounts available per capita, regardless of age, in a continuous series dating back to 1909.[8] Through the use of food composition tables, discussed below, USDA officials convert the foods available for consumption into nutrients and calories.

Such data, useful as they are, have their own reliability problems. Consider what might be involved in counting the pounds of carrots, corn, spinach, or beef produced in the United States each year, let alone the amounts imported or exported. Inevitably, some food is spoiled or wasted, but it is difficult to know how much. It is also difficult to know how much food is produced in home gardens (which would increase the per capita availability) or fed to pets (which would decrease it). Overall, food supply figures almost certainly overestimate food consumption. Indeed, per capita calorie availability since 2000 has amounted to 3,900 per day, nearly twice the FDA's 2,000-calorie standard. Since 1970 the USDA has addressed this overestimation by correcting calorie supply figures for wastage.[9] Wastage, according to the agency, now accounts for about 1,300 of the available 3,900 daily calories per capita.

TABLE 14   COMPARISON OF AVERAGE CALORIE INTAKE
(OR AVAILABILITY) PER PERSON PER DAY, DETERMINED BY
VARIOUS METHODS

Method	Men	Women	Population average
Doubly labeled water studies (measured calorie expenditure)	3,050	2,400	—
FDA calorie intake standard for food labels (selected for convenience)	—	—	2,000
What We Eat in America, 2008 (self-reported food intake)	2,500	1,800	2,070
Average of USDA dietary intake surveys prior to 1990 (self-reported food intake)	—	—	2,350
USDA calorie availability, corrected for waste, 2008 (food supply data)	—	—	2,670
USDA Beltsville study, 1984 (self-reported food intake)	2,760	1,850	—
USDA calorie availability, 2006 (food supply data)	—	—	3,900

CALORIE INTAKE PER DAY

At this point it is amusing to summarize the results of the various studies that have addressed the question of the number of calories the average American eats in a day and to compare them to the "gold standard" figures obtained from doubly labeled water experiments. We do this in table 14.

It isn't really fair to compare the numbers in this table, because they derive from studies using different methods on different groups of people, and some were measured, while others were self-reported or estimated. Nevertheless, we think this table illustrates some useful points:

+ Various methods for determining calorie intake produce widely varying results.
+ Measured values exceed self-reported values by 500 calories a day or more.
+ Food supply data corrected for waste come closest to measured calorie intake.
+ Only self-reported results come close to the FDA's 2,000-calorie-a-day standard.

Clearly, surveys of what Americans eat require cautious interpretation. Self-reported dietary intake tends to underestimate calorie consumption.

Food supply data tend to overestimate it. The truth lies someplace in between and, in any case, will vary among individuals and from day to day. Average calorie intake is likely to be close to the averages found with doubly labeled water studies but will be higher—sometimes much higher—among people who are gaining weight.

FOOD COMPOSITION TABLES

No matter what method is used to determine food intake, figuring out calorie intake means measuring the amounts of protein, fat, and carbohydrate—and sometimes alcohol—in the foods and drinks people consume and converting those amounts into calories. These kinds of laboratory analyses are cumbersome, costly, and time consuming, so most studies rely on the USDA's food composition tables, now published online as "National Nutrient Database for Standard Reference."[10] We consider this resource a national treasure. Every survey of dietary intake, every study of diet and health, and every determination of individual dietary intake depends on the USDA tables, with only rare exceptions.

With justifiable pride, the USDA boasts that it has produced data on the nutrient composition of American foods for more than one hundred years. Once again, this takes us back to Atwater who, after all, wrote his doctoral dissertation on the nutrient composition of corn. And in the late 1870s Atwater worked on the composition of seafood. In the early 1890s he and a colleague, C. D. Woods, published preliminary reports on the nutrient composition of about 200 foods and by 1896 had reported the amounts of protein, fat, carbohydrate, and calories in 2,600 foods.[11] Today the USDA provides analyses of calories and up to 142 distinct nutrient components in more than 7,500 different foods. Without question, these tables constitute the most authoritative and comprehensive source of information about the nutrient content of foods available anywhere.

Despite their incomparable worth, these tables—like almost everything about nutrition—are estimations and require cautious interpretation. Their calorie values still depend on the 1955 Modified Atwater Values. Look up the Nutrient Database entry for "cheese food, cold pack, American," for example. The calories listed for protein, fat, and carbohydrate are identical to those given for milk products in 1955. Is milk in 2011 identical to milk in 1955? We have no idea, especially if analytic methods have changed over time.

Other limitations have to do with variations in the growing conditions and varieties of foods. To determine the number of calories in, say, Georgia peanuts, you would need to select peanuts grown on a particular farm (Jimmy Carter's, for example), decide how many constitute a representative sample, and weigh the sample carefully. You would not typically burn the peanuts in a bomb calorimeter. Instead, you would analyze the grams of water, mineral matter (ash), protein, and fat, and assume the remainder is carbohydrate. You then estimate calories by multiplying the grams of each component by its Modified Atwater Value.

But are Jimmy Carter's peanuts the same as those grown elsewhere? The USDA nutrient data team must decide which peanuts are most likely to be representative, how large a sample to test, how many samples to analyze, and how many analyses to perform. They must deal with questions about sample collection and preservation and the reliability of analytical techniques. The analyses are expensive, but the USDA's budget for such studies is limited. This means that the USDA must rely not only on information provided by university scientists but also on analyses provided more or less voluntarily by food companies required to do such determinations as the basis for Nutrition Facts labels. But food companies are often reluctant to provide any additional information, even though they have it, as they consider nutrient composition to be proprietary information—another example of food politics in action.[12] Fortunately for our purposes, food companies have to list calories on food labels.

The makers of alcoholic beverages, however, do not. Beer, wine, and hard liquor are not regulated as foods, and the FDA has hardly anything to do with them. It is now time to discuss the calories in alcohol.

CHAPTER 11

Secret Calories

Alcohol

Until now we have ignored the contribution of alcohol to calorie intake, mainly because not everyone drinks spirits, wine, or beer. Also, alcohol is metabolized somewhat differently than the other energy-producing molecules in food. But beer, wine, and hard liquor most certainly provide calories. For the most part these calories are empty. Alcoholic beverages typically contain no nutrients or so few that they are hardly worth mentioning.[1]

THE SCIENCE AND POLITICS OF EARLY INVESTIGATIONS

For the discovery of the calorie value of alcohol, we must turn yet again to Wilbur Atwater. Until 1897 his publications of food composition did not list alcoholic beverages. That year, he and Charles Ford Langworthy reported the results of their analyses of the contribution of beer and other sources of alcohol calories to daily diets. In 1902 Atwater and Francis Benedict published a 166-page monograph devoted entirely to a thorough review of their own and other investigators' studies of alcoholic beverages as sources of food energy.[2]

This monograph is a good example of how quickly calories became enmeshed in politics. The title page cites its major source of funding as "The Committee of Fifty for the Investigation of the Drink Problem." Actually named the Committee of Fifty for the Investigation of the Liquor Problem, this was a private research group formed in 1893 to establish a scientific basis for policies to control alcohol use and abuse. Its members included bankers, economists, professors, and ethicists. The committee was not part of the religion-based Prohibition movement, aimed at banning all consumption of alcoholic beverages. Instead, its wealthy and educated members fretted about the need to maintain social order in the face of rising levels of alcohol abuse—especially among the working classes.[3]

With the backing of this group, Atwater and Benedict conducted at least thirty studies to determine the calorie value of alcohol. Some of these studies involved whole-body calorimeter experiments in which they gave volunteers, one at a time, as much alcohol "as they could well take without apparent nervous disturbance." Atwater and Benedict measured digestion, excretion, and metabolism as the men rested, read, or rode stationary bicycles during periods lasting up to four days.

The results were unambiguous. Healthy young men could absorb alcohol almost completely and use its energy just as they used energy from protein, fat, or carbohydrate. As a source of calories, alcohol behaved like any other food component. But this conclusion, Atwater and Benedict rightly suspected, would not be received well in certain circles: "Aside from the question of the power of alcohol to protect protein and fat and supply energy to the body for various useful purposes, there are the far weightier considerations of the general effect of alcohol upon the muscular and especially the nervous system and upon health and welfare. Upon these most serious hygienic, economical, and ethical problems the experiments here reported throw no special light."[4]

The investigators' explicit lack of attention to the "special light" appalled Prohibitionists. At the time, the burgeoning temperance movement was centered in the Methodist church. Atwater was the son of a Methodist minister and worked at Wesleyan, a university with close ties to the Methodist church. The church establishment viewed his work on alcohol calories as a disgrace to the religion. Atwater had to assure his fellow Methodists that he was not, in fact, recommending alcohol. He was simply observing that most people could consume it in moderation. For those who did, he said, alcohol appeared to improve their well-being, rather than to damage it.[5] It was not possible to keep his research free from the politics of religion in that era.

THE CALORIES IN ALCOHOL

Atwater and his colleagues took careful measurements of the fuel value of alcohol. In the bomb calorimeter, alcohol produced a gross energy value of 7.07 calories per gram. They could find no trace of excreted alcohol in feces, meaning that all of the consumed alcohol was absorbed. But, they observed, about 2 percent of the calories from ingested alcohol were lost from the lungs, skin, and kidneys. From their respiration calorimeter measurements, they concluded that 98 percent of alcohol calories were available to the body. Therefore, the energy from alcohol available to the body must be 6.9 calories per gram.

Seventy years later, USDA nutritionists took up what they called "the perplexing subject of the energy value of alcohol." The perplexity as they saw it derived from questions about the extent to which alcohol calories are actually available for use by the body. Their review of Atwater's and subsequent studies led them to conclude that 6.93 calories per gram is a more accurate value than Atwater's 1902 measurement of 6.9.[6]

In the early 2000s Geoffrey Livesey recalculated these values, taking the heat losses of metabolism into consideration. He proposed a net metabolizable energy value of 6.3 calories per gram for alcohol. As we discussed in chapter 7, international experts met in 2002 to develop a consensus about whether Atwater's calorie values should be revised. That group—which, you may recall, included Livesey—chose not to revise the alcohol value, mainly "because the problems and burdens ensuing from such a change would appear to outweigh by far the benefits." Instead, the group recommended the use of the rounded-off Atwater Value of 7.0 calories per gram.[7] Like the other Atwater Values, this one does not account for heat losses in metabolism.

The Atwater Value of 7 calories per gram underlies current USDA food composition tables for beer, wine, and hard liquor. These tables, however, do not specify alcohol as a nutrient. Instead, they give total calories and, when relevant, grams of carbohydrate (mostly sugars such as the maltose in beer), as shown in table 15.[8] By the USDA's definition, a standard serving of an alcoholic beverage contains 15 grams of pure alcohol, an amount that provides 105 calories as calculated from the Atwater Value of 7.0 calories per gram. For convenience, this gets rounded off to about 100 calories per serving, another one of those "good enough" estimations.

THE CALORIES IN ALCOHOLIC BEVERAGES

Beer, wine, and hard liquor do not necessarily come in standard servings. They are bottled to contain widely varying amounts of alcohol. Their calories are not always labeled, and it is not always easy to figure out how many calories they provide. This situation is grounded in history—and politics.

TABLE 15   CALORIES FROM ALCOHOL PROVIDED BY
STANDARD SERVINGS OF BEER, WINE, AND HARD LIQUOR

Beverage	Total calories	Calories from carbohydrate*	Calories from alcohol, by difference
Beer, 12 ounces†	150	50	100
Wine, 5 ounces	120	20	100
Gin, vodka, whisky, or rum, 80 proof, 1.5 ounces	100	0	100

NOTE: A standard serving contains 15 grams of pure alcohol.

*Calculated from grams of complex carbohydrates and sugars multiplied by the Atwater Value, 4 calories per gram. All figures rounded off.

†"Light" beer has less carbohydrate and, therefore, fewer calories.

Although alcoholic beverages provide calories and, therefore, qualify as food (just the way sugar does), they are not regulated as food. Instead, because of their tax-generating potential, the Treasury Department takes a special interest in these products through what it now calls the Alcohol and Tobacco Tax and Trade Bureau (TTB). The TTB regulates the content and labels of some—but not all—alcohol-containing drinks.

As we will explain further in chapter 24, the TTB regulations for labeling calories on alcoholic drinks, politically motivated as they are, border on the irrational. So do TTB rules for labeling alcohol percentage, from which calories can be calculated.[9] To summarize the TTB rules briefly:

- ✦ Distilled spirits must display percent alcohol by volume, but calorie disclosures are optional.
- ✦ Labels for wines containing 14 percent alcohol or more must display percent alcohol by volume; those below 14 percent alcohol may either disclose the percent or substitute a designation of type, such as table or light. Calories are optional.
- ✦ For regular beer, calorie levels and percent alcohol are optional.
- ✦ Labels of light beer must display calories but percent alcohol is optional.

The TTB regulates only these specific categories of alcoholic beverages. If a wine or hard cider contains less than 7 percent alcohol, it is regulated by the FDA. The FDA also has jurisdiction over any beer that is not made from barley and hops. Like all FDA-regulated foods, these drinks must display

Nutrition Facts labels that list calories. They may list the percentage of alcohol, but do not have to.

The result of the confusing rules for alcoholic beverage categories is that the labels of most wines and distilled spirits tell you practically nothing about nutrient contents. The only hints are statements of alcohol content, as percent alcohol by volume. Percent alcohol varies according to the drink: beer has 4–10 percent, wine 7–15 percent, champagne 8–14 percent, and distilled spirits 40–95 percent. Distilled spirits may list proof, which is twice the alcohol percent. Proof adds no new information but makes the alcohol level appear higher, a marketing strategy aimed at people who want more alcohol in their drinks.

Because molecules of alcohol are smaller than molecules of water, alcohol mixes with water and does not simply add to the volume of a drink. In the United States a standard alcohol beverage serving is considered to be a little more than half an ounce, or 18 milliliters (ml). A milliliter of water weighs 1 gram, but 1 milliliter of alcohol weighs about 0.8 gram.[10] That is why a standard serving of *alcohol* is considered to be about 15 grams, not 18. Grams, as always, are the basis of calorie determinations.

If you know the percent alcohol or the proof, you can figure out the calories in wine, regular beer, or hard liquor using the Atwater Value of 7 calories per gram. One ounce is a volume of 30 milliliters. Should you wish to try it, the formula goes like this:

$$\text{Percent alcohol} \times \text{number of ounces} \times 30 \text{ ml/ounce}$$
$$\times \: 0.8 \text{ gram/ml} \times 7 \text{ calories/gram}$$

Here's how this works: Suppose you have a bottle of wine labeled as 13.5 percent alcohol by volume. You pour six ounces into your glass—180 ml. Multiplying 180 by 0.135 gives you a bit more than 24 milliliters of alcohol. Multiply 24 by 0.8, and you have 19.2 grams of alcohol, which, when multiplied by 7 calories per gram, gives you about 135 calories. If you prefer to work from proof, you must divide that by 2 to get alcohol by volume.

This example began with a volume larger than the USDA standard serving size. Its calories are higher in proportion. Larger drinks have more calories, something that we wish were more obvious. For standard servings, it is reasonable to assume 100 calories per drink from the alcohol alone. For mixed drinks it is necessary to add any calories provided by the mixer (the sugary tonic water added to a gin and tonic, for example). You also have to include the additional calories from the sugars in wine or regular beer.

If you drink light beer, the labels do the calorie-counting work for you. The label of Pennsylvania's Yuengling Light Lager, for instance, gives an average analysis: 99 calories, 8.5 grams carbohydrates, 0.82 gram protein, and 0.1 gram fat. Forget about the protein and fat. Their calories are negligible. As with any "light" beer, a standard serving provides about 100 calories. But how much alcohol does it contain? You can figure this out by subtracting the minimal calories from protein, fat, and carbohydrate and working backward with the formula, but why bother? This is a light beer, and its percent alcohol will be closer to 4 percent than to 10 percent.

Nutrition advocacy groups have complained for years about the confusing and uninformative labeling of alcohol beverages and have pressed for a more rational system for displaying the content of alcohol, calories, and ingredients. But their efforts to date have not succeeded, as we explain in chapter 24.

DO ALCOHOL CALORIES COUNT?

Yes, they do. But if anything about alcohol calories can still be considered perplexing, it is surely the way they are metabolized in the body. Alcohol is not changed by digestion. It is absorbed into the body intact, where it goes straight to the liver. There enzymes convert it to acetaldehyde, a potentially toxic substance thought to be responsible for much of the damage to the liver, heart, and other organs seen so frequently in "heavy drinkers" who habitually drink too much alcohol.[11]

Unlike the way other energy-producing molecules in food are used in the body, how alcohol is metabolized depends greatly on the amount consumed. People who drink only small amounts of alcohol will readily metabolize acetaldehyde to acetate. Acetate enters normal energy-yielding metabolic pathways and ends up excreted as carbon dioxide and water or, if calories are in excess, stored as body fat. Large amounts of alcohol, however, increase the deposition of fat in the liver and overcome the body's ability to metabolize acetaldehyde. This substance accumulates and causes damage, especially to the liver and the heart. People vary greatly in the rates at which they metabolize alcohol, which is why it affects different people in such different ways.

These differences may explain why alcohol calories do not affect everyone's body weight in the same way. People who drink large amounts of alcohol are not necessarily more obese than nondrinkers and often display relatively lower body weights. This may be due to the substitution of alcohol for other sources of calories. Unless excessive alcohol intake has induced liver damage, so-called beer bellies are the result of excess calories from any source, not just beer.

Furthermore, the effects of alcohol seem to depend on levels of habitual drinking.[12] Among heavy—but not light—drinkers, alcohol has been shown to increase the amount of energy used in basal metabolism and in the thermic effects of metabolizing food. Whether this increase is due to liver damage, alcohol-induced impairment of metabolic pathways, or some other biochemical mechanism is as yet unknown. The key point here is this: if you are a social drinker who takes in relatively small amounts of alcohol, you are likely to use the calories in your alcohol drinks just as you would the calories from any other source. Alcohol calories count.

Although the ability to burn off alcohol calories as heat may be an effective weight-loss strategy for heavy drinkers, it is not one we recommend. Excessive alcohol intake irreparably damages the liver, and chronic alcohol users pay a high price in health and social costs for their reduced body weight.

CONSUMPTION OF ALCOHOL CALORIES IN THE UNITED STATES

The percentage of total daily calories contributed by alcohol varies according to the intake levels of a population, but intake can only be estimated, and not easily. Information about alcohol intake is even more susceptible to forgetting and evasion than information about food intake. Alcoholic drinks are taxable and, therefore, countable, but not all liquor consumed in this or any other country is legally produced. For 2008, the National Institute on Alcohol Abuse and Alcoholism estimated average alcohol consumption in the United States at 2.32 gallons of pure alcohol for every person age 14 or older, which calculates out to 135 calories per day from alcohol alone. But surveys have repeatedly reported that about one-third of the U.S. adult population does not drink alcohol at all. This means that alcohol calories are higher in light drinkers and much higher in heavy drinkers. In contrast to the consumption of food calories, consumption of alcohol has declined in the United States since 1980, when the per capita average was 2.76 gallons and 160 calories per day. Most of the decline is accounted for by reduced consumption of distilled spirits. Beer consumption also has decreased, but by a smaller amount, while the consumption of wine has remained about the same.[13]

CHAPTER 12

Calorie Regulation
The Body's Complex Weight Management System

A daily intake of more than 2,000 calories adds up to nearly a million calories a year, yet many people—without consciously doing anything about it—remain at about the same weight throughout their entire lives. Input and output can vary by hundreds of calories from day to day without causing any noticeable long-term change in body weight. Over time, something must be controlling calorie intake and balancing it against calorie expenditure with remarkable precision. But what?

How calorie regulation works is a question that thoroughly intrigues researchers, especially now that obesity has gone global. When discussing their work, scientists who study the regulation of body weight invariably invoke the same word: *complex.*[1] This requires translation. Whenever you hear scientists describe a biological phenomenon as complex, they are telling you that it is not well understood. And so it is with the regulation of calorie balance. Researchers have identified many biological components of the body weight regulatory system. They know a great deal about how complex the factors are but are just beginning to understand how regulatory factors operate and interact. The complexity leads scientists to suspect that the various factors, some with overlapping or as yet unidentified functions, evolved in order to keep bodies alive at times when food was scarce. In today's environment of food overabundance and widespread availability, these regulatory factors do not function nearly as well.

PHYSIOLOGICAL CONTROLS OF FOOD INTAKE

The need for food is so basic to life that a physiological system centered in the brain evolved to control it. To regulate eating behavior—hunger, the intake of food, and satiety—the brain responds to internal signals that tell it when more energy is needed and when it is not. Years ago, researchers found that they could induce laboratory animals to stop eating by destroying certain areas of their brains. By destroying other brain areas, they could stimulate the animals to eat excessively and grow fat.

Changes in levels of glucose or fatty acids in the blood—or the mere sight, smell, or taste of food—can affect perceptions of hunger or satiety. These perceptions signal the mouth, intestinal tract, fatty tissues, and other organs to release a multitude of hormones and other factors that affect the areas of the brain that control eating behavior. These factors tell the brain when the body needs to eat, how much to eat, and when to stop eating, and they also influence levels of spontaneous physical activity.[2] To illustrate why researchers consider food regulation complex, we list a small selection of these factors in table 16.

Most of the factors listed in this table inhibit the desire to eat and induce satiety after a meal. They interact with the nervous system in the intestine or communicate directly with the brain centers that influence feeding behavior. The mere presence of food and its digestive products in the stomach and intestine is all it takes to turn on secretion of some of these factors. Though these factors appear to be stop signals that modulate the consumption of individual meals, their role in longer-term regulation of energy stores is less certain.

Several intestinal factors stimulate the release of insulin by the pancreas. The pancreas also releases insulin in response to nutrients that enter the bloodstream, especially the sugar glucose. Insulin stimulates the metabolism and cellular storage of glucose, fatty acids, and amino acids after a meal and acts on the brain to inhibit food intake, but its action is complex (that word again, still indicating incomplete understanding). When levels of blood glucose decrease, people become hungry.

Another pancreatic hormone, glucagon, stimulates the release of glucose from liver glycogen to the bloodstream in response to low blood glucose levels. The interaction of insulin and glucagon keeps blood glucose levels high enough to fuel the brain but within ranges considered normal. Diabetes is

TABLE 16 SELECTED FACTORS IDENTIFIED AS PARTICIPATING IN
THE REGULATION OF FOOD INTAKE

Hormonal factor	Source	Effect on hunger	Selected examples of actions*
Ghrelin	Stomach	Increases	Signals brain feeding centers; stimulates growth hormone secretion
Cholecystokinin	Intestine	Decreases	Stimulates gall bladder contraction and pancreatic enzyme secretion
Glucagon-like peptide-1	Intestine	Decreases	Reduces blood glucose levels; delays stomach emptying
Glucagon-like peptide-2	Intestine	Decreases	Stimulates intestinal cell growth
Peptide YY	Intestine	Decreases	Delays stomach emptying
Oxyntomodulin	Colon	Decreases	Suppresses appetite
Amylin	Pancreas	Decreases	Reduces blood glucose levels
Glucagon	Pancreas	Decreases	Stimulates insulin secretion; stimulates glycogen breakdown; raises blood glucose levels
Insulin	Pancreas	Decreases	Reduces blood glucose levels; stimulates glycogen synthesis
Pancreatic polypeptide	Pancreas	Decreases	Stimulates stomach emptying; inhibits gallbladder activity
Leptin	Fatty tissues	Decreases	Regulates energy balance

SOURCE: Adapted from Suzuki et al., 2010:362 (see note 2).
*Hormones usually have multiple physiological actions, not all of which are listed here.

characterized by elevated levels of blood glucose. In type 1 diabetes, the pancreas fails to secrete insulin. In type 2 diabetes, the kind related to obesity, the pancreas secretes insulin but body cells resist its action and do not respond.

The cellular receptors and neurons in the brain that respond to hormonal and other signals mediate the control of calorie intake, satiety, and body weight. And social behavior, psychological state, culture, and the food environment influence both signals and receptors. One such factor is cigarette smoking. Some people who quit smoking gain weight rapidly, as much as 10 to 25 pounds. Research suggests that nicotine may suppress appetite by interacting with the receptors and neurons in the brain that are involved in food intake. When people stop smoking, feeding behavior is no longer inhibited and they increase calorie intake and gain weight.[3] Overall, the physiological signals that govern food intake and body weight are numerous, interconnected, and overlapping. This makes them exceedingly difficult to study or understand, singly or together. Hence: complex.

We have been following research on the control of calorie balance for decades. During this time we have watched researchers pounce on one signaling factor after another as *the* critical regulator of food intake and body weight. Their enthusiasm is understandable. If a drug could be found to mimic the action of a hormone that turned off hunger, it could help solve the obesity problem, and billions of people would buy it.

Pharmaceutical companies are working long and hard to find such drugs, but the complexity of the regulatory system explains why none found to date seems to work very well. Getting glucose to the brain is so critical that it is the regulatory system's first priority. To protect brain fuel supplies, the system evolved to be highly redundant. If one signaling factor fails to function, another quickly compensates. And because some signaling factors have multiple effects, drugs aimed at one function may also cause undesirable effects on others.

All of this means that no one signal is likely to be able to control energy balance on its own—not insulin, not glucagon, and not even ghrelin or leptin, two hormonal factors of much current interest. Ghrelin, secreted by the stomach and the duodenum, stimulates food intake. Leptin, released from fat tissue, indicates the state of long-term energy stores and appears to be an "eat less" signal.

Ghrelin

Ghrelin is the one factor in table 16 that stimulates hunger directly, whereas the others seem to stimulate hunger by their absence. It also stimulates gastric acid secretion, the secretion of hormones from the pancreas, and intestinal motility.[4] Blood levels of ghrelin increase before eating and during hunger, fasting, and weight loss. Levels fall after eating. When human volunteers are given an appropriate dose of ghrelin and presented with a buffet of foods, they tend to eat more than they would without the drug. Ghrelin gets its name from "growth hormone–releasing" peptide because it also stimulates the release of growth hormone. Whether growth hormone has anything to do with the regulation of hunger is uncertain.

A more relevant question is whether turning off ghrelin might also turn off hunger. Scientists have developed vaccines against ghrelin that do indeed cause rats and pigs to eat less and lose weight.[5] This approach may seem promising, but neither its applicability to humans nor its long-term consequences are known. Perhaps ghrelin is only involved in telling the body when to start and when to stop eating. We expect it will take some time before researchers find out whether ghrelin has a role in regulating long-term energy balance.

Leptin

Leptin, however, is almost certainly involved in the long-term regulation of body weight. It signals the brain about how much fat is available to the body. In groundbreaking work in the 1990s, Jeffrey Friedman and his colleagues discovered leptin, which they named after the Greek *leptos*, meaning "thin," through experiments with laboratory strains of genetically obese mice. Some of these strains have a defective gene for making leptin. Others have a defect in a brain receptor for the hormone. Without a working receptor, the brain cannot respond to leptin, even when the hormone's levels are high. Leptin has been found in the blood of all mammals studied to date, and all respond to it in the same way. When leptin levels are high, the animals eat less. When levels are low, the animals eat more.[6]

Do obese humans lack leptin? Indeed some do, but leptin deficiency turns out to be extremely rare in humans, obese or not. Friedman had to search the world to find a handful of people with genetic defects in leptin production similar to those in obese mice. Like the mice, these rare people also eat excessively and are extremely obese. But when they are treated with injections of leptin, their eating behavior returns to normal and they lose weight.

This promising result suggested that leptin could be the magic drug to help overweight people control their food intake. But alas, the results of the early leptin therapy trials have proved disappointing. When people reduce calorie intake, their blood levels of leptin fall, and they feel hungry. Perhaps the main function of leptin is to indicate when fat stores are reduced, signaling the body to eat. In that case, leptin supplements will not help restrain energy intake to any appreciable extent in most people.[7]

Some obese individuals display high levels of blood leptin but experience little or no restraint on food intake. Could they have defects in their leptin receptors? If so, finding a drug to prevent leptin resistance could be another promising research area.[8] Although research is ongoing, leptin shows few signs of alleviating all but the rarest forms of human obesity. As we keep saying, body weight regulation is complex.

HOW PRECISE IS THE BIOLOGICAL CONTROL
OF ENERGY BALANCE?

In the short term, the regulation of food intake is imprecise. If you fast today, you may or may not compensate for the calorie gap in the next few days. If you snack throughout the day, you may or may not eat fewer calories at subsequent meals. Despite this variation, the body weights of most people, even those who are overweight, reach a point of relative stability. This observation suggests that people might have a "set point" for energy storage—a specific weight, give or take a few pounds, that is strongly defended by physiological signals.[9]

Despite ongoing interest in this idea among writers of popular diet books, many obesity researchers now prefer to explain the observation as the expression of a "settling zone," a *range* of body weight, albeit relatively narrow, with upper and lower limits determined by genetics and other physiological variables that can be influenced by the food environment—the availability of food, its ease of access, and the ways in which it is marketed.[10] Because the lower limit of a body weight settling zone is more critical to survival than the upper limit, the lower limit is most heavily defended by biological signals. In this view, the amount of body fat does not need to be controlled very carefully by internal signals. Instead, body fat serves as a depository for excessive calories that accumulate as a result of errors in the control of food intake.

WHAT ABOUT GENETICS?

The example of leptin suggests that the genes involved in control of calorie intake, calorie expenditure, and energy balance could be likely to influence body weight. Some researchers believe that genetic factors account for 40 to 70 percent of the variation in body weight in human populations—an enormous percentage in biological terms. Others think such percentages are greatly exaggerated in the face of today's "eat more" food environment, in which tasty, relatively inexpensive food is readily available and heavily marketed to encourage frequent eating of large amounts (see chapter 21). Genetics, after all, cannot have changed since 1980, when rates of obesity began to rise.

Occasionally, as with the rare cases of leptin deficiency, investigators do find defects in single genes associated with obesity. One study of about 2,200 severely obese children identified 7 percent with identifiable defects in single genes.[11] But most cases of obesity are far more complex (again, that word). They appear to involve multiple genes that interact to influence responses to the food environment. Still, because not everyone in today's food environment becomes obese, it makes sense to believe that some people are more genetically susceptible to environmental influences than others.

Some scientists believe that the high current levels of obesity can be explained by "thrifty genes."[12] The thinking behind this attractive—but as yet unproven—hypothesis begins with the idea that ancient humans experienced frequent periods of famine as a result of extremes in climate and, later, of crop failures. When food was plentiful, genetically determined imperatives to eat as many calories and to store as much body fat as possible made biological sense. People who stored the most energy in times of plenty could survive famine, reproduce more efficiently, and pass on their genes to a new generation. But when food is abundant, these genetic determinants cause people to overeat.

Studies of Pima Indians living on an Arizona reservation are often cited as evidence for the interaction of thrifty genes with diet and activity patterns.[13] In the later decades of the twentieth century, the Pima began to display exceptionally high rates of obesity and type 2 diabetes. This change was almost certainly the result of switching from traditional diets and hunting-and-gathering lifestyles to those more typical of modern, industrialized America. In comparison, groups of genetically similar Pima Indians living more traditionally in remote mountainous areas of Mexico have not become overweight and display lower rates of diabetes.

Attractive as it is, the idea of thrifty genes is not universally accepted. If such genes were so important for the survival of ancient humans, then everyone living in modern-day "eat more" food environments ought to be obese. John Speakman, a biologist from Aberdeen, views obesity in modern society more as a matter of "genetic drift." By this he means that ancient conditions of intermittent semistarvation led to strong selection pressures against low levels of body fat. Fewer such pressures promoted limits on the overall amount of body fat. These unequal selection pressures and random gene mutations led to an increase in the upper limit of the settling zone for some people, thereby allowing them to store larger amounts of body fat. Placed in an environment where food is plentiful and sensory stimuli are strong, such individuals become obese. Speakman calls this idea the "drifty gene" hypothesis.[14]

Regardless of the mechanism through which they operate, genetic theories of obesity can never be simple. More than one hundred genes have been identified as having some effect on body weight. The Rockefeller University obesity researcher Rudolf Leibel argues that these genes act primarily through the central nervous system and affect both conscious and unconscious aspects of food intake and energy expenditure. No regulatory gene, acting alone or in concert with others, can explain the risk of becoming obese, in part because its expression depends so much on its interaction with other genes as well as with the food environment.[15]

BIOLOGY VS. THE FOOD ENVIRONMENT

Jeffrey Friedman argues compellingly for a biological basis for obesity. He notes that while dieters can consciously override the basic drive to eat for short periods of time, most cannot keep doing so. Hormones such as leptin and ghrelin that stimulate appetite after weight loss do not adapt quickly to reduced body weight. They continue to send out "eat more" signals for as much as a year after weight loss. Eventually, biology wins out. "The world would be a better place," Friedman says, "if people who deride the obese kept this in mind."[16]

The consequence of having dozens of genes involved in body weight regulation is that you are likely to have a hard time controlling your calorie balance. The urge to eat is so fundamental to life that multiple overlapping and powerful regulatory factors evolved to maintain that urge and to prompt you to eat as much as you can at every opportunity. When you are exposed to the pleasures of highly palatable food and the marketing that promotes its frequent consumption, your much weaker regulatory stop signals are easily overcome.

Dr. David Kessler, a former FDA commissioner, expands on this idea in his book *The End of Overeating*. The food environment, he argues, provides so much food designed deliberately to excite pleasure centers that it overrides biological stop signals. The factors that discourage calorie intake and promote satiety ought to function quite well in environments that encourage the consumption of diets high in nutrient density and low in calorie density. But in food environments that aggressively promote overconsumption of high-calorie foods, the "eat more" signals overpower those that promote satiety. In such environments, matters largely beyond personal control— the presence of other people, the location of meals, how often meals appear, how large food portions might be, how tasty the foods are, and how they are advertised—are remarkably effective at overcoming physiological regulatory mechanisms.[17]

With this regulatory imbalance in mind, let's take a look at how the system works in practice to protect vital body functions during periods of extreme fasting or forced starvation. At both extremes—too few and too many calories—the regulatory system compensates well for relatively small day-to-day differences in intake and expenditure. This means that losing or gaining weight requires the habitual intake of calories below or above normal maintenance levels, a subject we consider in chapter 17.

PART FOUR

Too Few Calories

People do not usually choose to eat too few calories to support their energy needs. When they do, they feel hungry. The pangs of hunger are acute enough to make anyone want to eat, and right away. Chronic hunger is most often forced upon people by poverty, war, or natural disasters. But sometimes people who have plenty of food available choose not to eat. They diet to lose weight. They fast for religious or political reasons. Or they deliberately restrict calorie intake in an attempt to live longer. In this part of the book we zero in on the physiological and some of the political implications of inadequate calorie intake, whether forced or voluntary. Because the biology of calorie deprivation is the same no matter what its cause, we consider both the forced and the more acute voluntary situations together. Our discussion of dieting, usually a temporary and milder form of calorie deprivation, comes later, in part 5. If you want to understand why so many people find dieting difficult and why dieting so rarely succeeds, it helps to understand the body's response to consuming too few calories.

The effects of inadequate calorie intake are not limited to unpleasant sensations. Hunger is at first accompanied by loss of weight, muscle strength, alertness, and stamina and later by increasing impairment of all body functions. If deprivation is severe enough, it leads to death. These effects are more severe in young children, who have proportionately greater needs for calories and nutrients than adults do. Undernourished children do not grow properly. They become depressed, irritable, and apathetic. They do not learn well in school. Their immune systems fail, making them more susceptible to the hazards of microbial infections, especially diarrhea and its accompanying losses of nutrients. Infections, in turn, increase caloric requirements. The repeated cycle of too few calories, infections, and increased calorie needs is the principal immediate cause of death among many young children in many parts of the world, even today. Its underlying causes, of course, are political: social and income inequality or instability. Worldwide hunger among both children and adults is the most acute situation in which the science and politics of calorie availability are inextricably linked.

We begin our discussion of such issues with an examination of the biological consequences of extreme caloric restriction, no matter what its cause.

CHAPTER 13

Starvation and Its Effects on the Body

The immediate response to a need for more calories is hunger for food. Feelings of hunger may be mild or intense and can range from slight irritation to extreme agony. Chronic hunger is a miserable experience, but the degree to which it induces mental misery depends greatly on whether the calorie deprivation is voluntary or forced. Although people with plenty of access to food may say "I'm starving" when they haven't eaten for a few hours, the difference between voluntary and forced hunger is so critical that scientific publications and newspaper articles often describe them in different words. *Fasting* refers to voluntary calorie deprivation, while the forced situations are called *starvation* or *semistarvation*.

Regardless of what they call it, scientists know exactly what calorie deprivation does to human physiology and psychology. The effects depend entirely on how long the deprivation lasts and how extreme it is. People may feel hungry during the daylong fasts of Yom Kippur and Ramadan or longer "cleansing" fasts, but such short periods of deprivation rarely induce lasting harm. Once people start eating again, they quickly make up for the missing calories.

Forced starvation, however, is deadly, and scientists know all too much about it. Over the years, they have repeatedly documented the effects of starvation, and in excruciating detail. During World War II, for example, a group of Jewish doctors meticulously recorded the effects of food deprivation on people imprisoned behind the walls of the Warsaw Ghetto, even going so far as to document the physiological signs of their own decline.[1] Case studies of fasting individuals occasionally appear in medical journals. One described the physiological effects of a forty-day total fast undertaken under medical supervision by a cloistered member of a religious community (we show what happened to his body weight in figure 12 on page 119).[2]

People who are obese and have large stores of body fat can remain alive for many months without eating. But people who are thin cannot. This difference also has been well researched and is especially known through accounts of hunger strikers who voluntarily refused food in order to achieve political goals. When people who are not obese consume nothing but water, they are able to survive for a remarkably consistent two months, give or take a week or so.

In 1981, for example, ten men imprisoned in Northern Ireland starved themselves to death as an act of political protest. Their leader, Bobby Sands, stopped eating on March 1; he died 66 days later, on May 5. For the ten hunger strikers, the average time to death was 62 days, with a range of 46 to 73 days. Make no mistake: these were not easy deaths. As was evident from communications smuggled out of the prison, extreme calorie deprivation—even when voluntary—induces extreme physical suffering.[3]

ANCEL KEYS'S STUDIES OF SEMISTARVATION

Even less extreme calorie deprivation is difficult to endure. This also is well known, not least from the extraordinary experiment in human semistarvation conducted by the Minnesota cardiologist Ancel Keys toward the end of World War II. In 1944 Keys and his colleagues convinced a large group of church, foundation, university, and government sponsors to fund a study of semistarvation. Its purpose would be to help understand how prisoners and ordinary citizens might respond to adverse food conditions such as those expected in Europe at the close of the war and how to rehabilitate those who were starving.

The investigators recruited 32 conscientious objectors—all young, lean, and healthy men—who volunteered to lose 25 percent of their body weight in six months while under close observation and monitoring. Keys and his colleagues, in a 1950 monograph reminiscent of the prodigious output of Wilbur Atwater, published the results of these investigations in two volumes of more than 700 pages each.[4]

To induce weight loss, the investigators allowed the volunteers to eat about 1,600 calories a day in the form of a bland diet largely based on potatoes, designed to mimic what might be expected to be available in concentration camps under wartime conditions. In order to make sure that the men lost 25 percent of their initial body weights, the researchers reduced the already restricted calorie allowance even further over the course of the study. After six months the men had indeed lost a quarter of their initial body weights. A *Life* magazine photograph of five of them lying shirtless on the grass is a shocking sight. The men were emaciated, with prominent ribs and wasted muscles. Although they were mostly in their twenties, they looked middle-aged.[5]

This study examined every conceivable aspect of the physiology and behavior of the semistarved men in astonishing detail. To summarize:

- Basal metabolic rates declined by about 25 percent.
- Body weights fell rapidly during the first two or three weeks of food deprivation, by a pound or two a day. Weight loss then tapered off to one or two pounds a week.
- Body fat levels declined, but so did the size of all muscles and body organs.
- Bones and teeth were not affected. The men showed no signs of vitamin or mineral deficiencies.
- The men's skin became pallid and cold to the touch.
- Their muscles became weaker, their endurance declined precipitously, and they reduced all unnecessary movement.
- They became lethargic, depressed, irritable, cold, and uninterested in sex but thoroughly obsessed with thoughts of food.

Some of these findings were expected. Calorie restriction was already well known to reduce the basal metabolism, thermic effect of food, and total energy expenditure of experimental animals. But other findings—the absence of vitamin and mineral deficiencies, for example—seem surprising. They are explained in part by the conditions of this experiment. The men had access to clean beds, hot showers, and soap, and the diet, uninteresting as it might have been, was balanced in nutrients. As body fat and muscles depleted, they released vitamins and minerals that could be used to keep other organs functioning. Keys stopped the experiment before permanent damage occurred, and the men eventually recovered from their ordeal. Decades later they were proud to have participated in a study that produced so much information about how the human body responds to calorie deprivation.[6]

THE PHYSIOLOGY OF CALORIE DEPRIVATION

Bodies do not like being denied food. There is a good reason why hunger is so unpleasant. If you are deprived of calories, you want food, and you want it *now*. The Minnesota experiment makes sense from the standpoint of the thrifty-gene or the drifty-gene hypotheses. Humans evolved to survive when food was scarce. Times of deprivation may have been difficult, but they were survivable, and for years. Survival of semistarvation is possible because human physiology adjusts—and quickly—to compensate for inadequate food energy.

From the standpoint of physiology, hunger is an emergency. The brain requires glucose—the sugar in blood—as fuel. Its need for about 100 grams of glucose a day (nearly a quarter of a pound) is a metabolic priority. Normal mixed diets contain enough carbohydrate to meet this need easily. Hunger is the first sign that the amount of glucose in blood may not be enough to keep the brain functioning. If hunger continues, the balance of regulatory hormones shifts to ensure that blood is continually supplied with adequate amounts of fuel—even when dietary carbohydrates are inadequate or absent. During prolonged calorie deficits, hormone levels shift even further to protect protein stores and preserve vital body enzymes, muscles, and organs as well as to reduce the body's energy requirements.

As we discussed in chapter 12, these processes involve the actions and interactions of many hormonal regulatory factors. In the absence of adequate calories, blood glucose levels fall, and the balance of hormones shifts to cause body stores of carbohydrate (liver and muscle glycogen), protein (muscles), and fat to break down into their constituent molecules—glucose, amino acids, and fatty acids—which can be metabolized for energy.

It is easiest to explain what happens during food deprivation by separating its effects into stages of *acute* starvation, when people take in nothing except water. The stages overlap considerably, and the times given are approximate. The duration of each stage depends on the proportion of energy needs met by food intake. In semistarvation, when people get some food but not enough to meet energy needs, the stages are prolonged. The Minnesota experiment, for example, gave the volunteers just barely enough food to maintain them in reasonable health while they were semistarved. If the men were not losing weight rapidly enough, the investigators reduced their rations.

First Few Hours: Glycogen Breaks Down to Glucose

When you are asleep and not eating, your brain still needs glucose. Enzymes break down the glycogen in your liver to glucose. The liver usually stores enough glycogen to take care of glucose needs for relatively short periods of fasting—while you are sleeping, for example.

Overnight or during the First Day: Depletion of Liver and Muscle Glycogen

Once liver glycogen is well on its way to depletion, the regulatory system goes into action, and the balance of hormones shifts to promote disassembly of the glycogen in muscles. Body proteins and fats break down to amino acids and fatty acids to be used for energy (see chapter 5). This process also releases the parts of amino acids and the glycerol part of fat that can be used to make glucose. Because glycogen binds up to four times its weight in water, its breakdown releases that water. On average, people store a pound or more of glycogen in muscles and liver.[7] The immediate weight loss that occurs with brief periods of fasting can be accounted for by the loss of glycogen and its associated bound water.

First Few Days: Breakdown of Body Proteins and Fats

As the total fast continues, hormonal shifts become more pronounced. They signal body proteins and fats to break down more quickly to produce amino acids and glycerol that can be used to make glucose. They also signal the kidneys to excrete salt. The excretion of salt is accompanied by the excretion of water, which is another reason why early weight loss occurs so rapidly. People who are fasting can lose a pound or two a day during this period, but most of the loss is explained by excreted water.

After Several Days: Ketones Replace Glucose as Fuel for the Brain

The increasingly rapid breakdown of body proteins to provide the makings of blood glucose cannot go on for long without destroying muscle and enzyme function and causing serious harm. To preserve life, vital body proteins must be conserved. But so must fuel for the brain. Here we have a physiological dilemma. Most of the stored energy in the body is in the form of fat. Fat

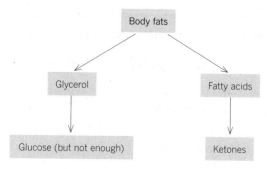

FIGURE 11. Synthesis of ketones. When blood glucose levels are low for several days, body fats break down so quickly that fatty acids are converted to ketones. Ketones substitute for glucose as fuel for the brain.

triglycerides break down to fatty acids just as rapidly as protein breaks down to amino acids, but except for their glycerol portion, triglycerides cannot be used to make glucose. Neither can the fatty acids. Glycerol converts rapidly to a compound that can be used to make glucose (two glycerols form one molecule of glucose). But the amount of glucose that can be made from the glycerol part of fat is not nearly enough to meet the brain's daily energy requirements, even when combined with the glucose made from parts of disassembled amino acids.

This unfortunate problem—you can make fat from glucose, but you can't make enough glucose from fat—has a solution. When blood glucose is falling and fat is breaking down rapidly, the metabolic reactions that produce energy are too slow to keep up with the influx of fatty acids released from the breakdown of fat. The reactions are swamped with surplus fatty acids. To relieve these metabolic pressures, enzymes in the liver and kidney convert the surplus fatty acids into compounds called ketones. As ketone levels rise in blood, the brain gradually adapts to using them for fuel. This process is shown in figure 11.

After a Week or So: Conservation of Body Proteins

Once the brain substitutes ketones for glucose, the breakdown of body fat becomes the primary source of energy. Body proteins also continue to break down, but more gradually, thereby conserving vital muscle functions such as those of the heart and diaphragm (the muscle that controls breathing). The intestinal tract, having nothing to do, begins to shed its lining of villi, the

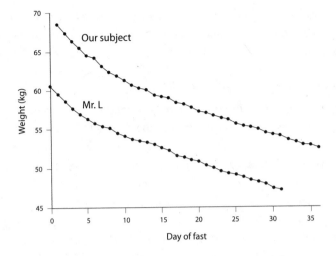

FIGURE 12. Rate of weight loss in two men who consumed nothing but water for a month or more. Their weights declined by 0.9 kg (about 2 pounds) per day for the first five days, then weight loss decreased gradually over the next two weeks and stabilized at a rate of 0.3 kg (about 0.7 pound) per day after the third week. "Our subject" was a monk fasting under the supervision of Kerndt and his colleagues in 1982, who compared his rate of weight loss to that of "Mr. L," as reported by Francis Benedict in 1915. Although the initial weights of the men differed by 20 pounds, the rates of weight loss were much the same. Source: Kerndt et al., 1982:382 (see note 2).

cellular structures where digestion and absorption take place. This leads to further weight loss. At this stage, weight loss increasingly reflects losses of body fat and protein. Physiologists have measured the rate of weight loss in total starvation, as shown in figure 12.

After One to Three Weeks: Reduction in Basal Metabolic Rate

The weight loss—and the continued shifts in the balance of hormones—slows down the body's energy requirements. The result is that it takes less energy to support body functions. The basal metabolic rate drops in direct proportion to the loss in body weight. Weight loss slows. Most of the weight loss derives from body fat, but small amounts of protein continue to be lost from all organs. In prolonged semistarvation, blood pressure falls, and people feel nauseated, become dizzy when they stand up, and do everything they can to avoid unnecessary movement. The Minnesota volunteers, for example, were deeply lethargic and could barely manage the tasks they were assigned. Few voluntary fasts last beyond this stage, as the risk of death increases rapidly from then on.

After Four Weeks or So: Depletion of Body Fat

Fasting or starvation can go on for only so long. At some point—sooner in leaner people but later in people with more body fat—fat stores run out and body proteins are all that remain to draw on for body energy and brain fuel. Once that stage is reached, all body systems collapse. The Irish hunger strikers became dangerously ill. Their wounds would not heal. They became blind and delirious. Eventually, they lapsed into coma. Once the heart and diaphragm muscles become weak, starving people are no longer able to clear fluids from the lungs. This makes them increasingly susceptible to lung infection, explaining why pneumonia is so often the cause of death of undernourished people.

RECOVERY FROM STARVATION

One relatively early effect of calorie deprivation is the reduction in size and complexity of the lining of the digestive tract. Ordinarily it is lined with villi, tiny threads of cells that produce digestive enzymes. These form a thick carpet with an enormous surface area for digesting and absorbing nutrients. Villi are especially sensitive to food deprivation. Without food, they atrophy and stop producing digestive enzymes. This reduces the surface area of the entire length of the digestive tract, making it increasingly difficult to absorb food molecules.

Starving people cannot digest or absorb food very well. If they eat beyond the absorptive capacity of the intestine, unabsorbed molecules pass into the large intestine, where bacteria ferment them, producing gas and diarrhea. Refeeding must take place slowly and gradually until the intestinal tract is fully functional. Even when permitted to consume thousands of extra calories a day, the men in the Minnesota experiment took many weeks to gain back the weight they had lost. They had much repairing to do.

CHAPTER 14

Individuals, Communities, Nations

Calories and Global Hunger

Late in 2010 the United Nations' Food and Agriculture Organization (FAO) announced what passes for good news on the international scene. By its estimation, "only" about 925 million people throughout the world were suffering from chronic hunger. This number, enormous as it is, represented a decline of nearly 10 percent from the previous year.[1]

How did the FAO arrive at this count? In a word, calories.

To make such estimates, the FAO asks each of its 192 member countries to provide three kinds of statistical information:

+ The amounts of all food commodities produced, used for seed and animal feed, wasted, imported, and exported. From these data and the calorie content of each food, the FAO estimates the total *availability of calories* for human consumption within each country.

+ The distribution of men and women in the population, by age. The FAO uses this information to estimate the country's *total calorie requirements*.

+ Household food surveys. These permit the FAO to estimate the *distribution of calories* available within the country.[2]

With this collection of data, the FAO can estimate the number of people in each country likely to meet its criterion for defining someone as chronically undernourished and hungry: consuming fewer than 1,800 calories per day. By FAO standards, this is the minimum calorie intake needed to maintain light activity. To arrive at the worldwide total, the FAO sums up the number of people who are consuming fewer than 1,800 calories a day in its member countries and regions, as shown in table 17.

TABLE 17   REGIONAL DISTRIBUTION OF BELOW-MINIMUM
CALORIE INTAKE, 2010

Region of the world	Millions of people consuming fewer than 1,800 calories per day
Asia and the Pacific	578
Sub-Saharan Africa	239
Latin America and the Caribbean	53
Near East and North Africa	37
Industrialized countries	19
Total	926

SOURCE: FAO, 2010 (see note 1).

These totals are based on statistical information provided by each country, but the collection of such data involves many potential sources of error. Countries vary in their ability to produce any statistical data at all, let alone accurate reports of food availability and use. The numbers submitted to the FAO may well be influenced by political considerations of whether it is in a country's best interest to appear to have adequate food available or to have a greater proportion of its population undernourished. The FAO numbers cannot be taken at face value but must be understood as a rough approximation of the state of food insecurity in the world. Regardless of their accuracy, FAO estimates emphasize that habitual intake of calories below expenditure makes it difficult, if not impossible, to maintain a healthy body weight or support "economically necessary and socially desirable physical activity."[3]

The FAO first published hunger estimates based on this method for the years 1969–71. Because this method differs from those of previous years, earlier data are not comparable. In the early 1970s the FAO estimated that 878 million people were chronically hungry, and the count has remained well above 800 million ever since. But because the world population has grown, the percentage of malnourished people has declined by the FAO's definition. That constitutes the extent of the good news.

UNEQUAL CALORIE DISTRIBUTION

Although the FAO uses calories as a convenient measure of hunger, nutritional health is not—and never can be—just about calories. Food variety and quality also matter. This key point is illustrated by the "Food Balance Sheets"

TABLE 18   CALORIES AVAILABLE IN THE FOOD SUPPLIES OF
SELECTED COUNTRIES AND REGIONS, PER PERSON PER DAY

Country or region	Total food calories	Plant-source calories	Animal-source calories
United States	3,750	2,720	1,030
Southern Europe	3,410	2,490	920
Australia, New Zealand	3,220	2,150	1,070
Oceana	3,180	2,160	1,020
Central America	3,040	2,470	570
Asia	2,670	2,270	400
Africa	2,455	2,270	185
East Africa	2,045	1,900	145
Eritrea	1,605	1,535	70
Entire world	2,795	2,315	480

SOURCE: FAO, 2007 (see note 4).
NOTE: Calories are rounded off to the nearest 5.

produced by the FAO. These are detailed tables of food and calorie availability presented separately for each member nation and region.[4] Food balance sheets present the total food calories available per person per day but also the number of calories derived from plant foods (fruit, vegetables, grains, beans) and animal foods (meat, dairy, eggs). Table 18 shows some examples of this distribution in 2007.

The world produces nearly 2,800 calories from food each day for every person of any age, which ought to be more than enough to feed everyone adequately. But the distribution of these calories is anything but equal. By the FAO's count, the United States has the largest number of calories available for its population, 3,750 per person per day (the USDA's figure is 3,900). In sharp contrast, the FAO estimates that Eritrea, in sub-Saharan Africa, has only 1,605 calories available per person per day. In the United States, as we discuss below, 15 percent of the population is considered "food insecure" but not necessarily hungry or undernourished. In contrast, the FAO deems 75 percent of the Eritrean population to be chronically deprived of food.

The calorie figures provide one other index of unequal food distribution: the relative proportion of calories from plant and animal sources. Although it is quite possible to consume a nutritionally adequate diet based entirely on plant foods, the inclusion of some foods from animal sources increases variety and adds nutrients that may be low or lacking in food plants. Foods from animals provide one vitamin—vitamin B_{12}—that is entirely lacking in plants along with higher amounts of protein, iron, zinc, and several other B vitamins. Young children in developing countries whose diets include small amounts of animal foods thrive better than those whose diets do not.[5] Countries display more than tenfold disparities in the number of calories available from animal foods, ranging from only 70 per capita per day in Eritrea to more than 1,000 in the most industrialized countries. As we emphasize repeatedly, calories alone cannot indicate the quality of diets, but they do provide a measure of the overall availability and variety of food.

PROTEIN VS. CALORIES

No matter how it is defined, chronic malnutrition—or, more precisely, undernutrition, the acute or chronic result of inadequate food, calories, and nutrients—has devastating effects, especially on young children. Chronic calorie deprivation induces the effects of semistarvation, described in the previous chapter. And when the diets they consume are severely limited in food variety, children may experience nutrient deficiencies, most commonly of vitamin A, iodine, iron, and zinc. Undernourished children are prone to diarrheal and other infectious diseases that further deplete their nutrient stores and increase calorie requirements. Unless the deprivation is reversed, death rates among undernourished children can be high.

These consequences have stimulated much research aimed at identifying simple nutritional solutions to malnutrition. Cicely Williams, a pediatrician working in West Africa in the early 1930s, is credited with some of the earliest attempts. She observed a childhood condition referred to in the language of the Gold Coast, now Ghana, as *kwashiorkor*, the "disease of the displaced child." Children developed the swollen bellies of kwashiorkor when their mothers weaned them in order to breastfeed a new baby.

Dr. Williams suspected that this disease was caused by the nutritionally inadequate corn-gruel diet given to infants after they were weaned. Although many of the symptoms she observed reflected what we now understand as an overall deficiency of calories and the full range of essential nutrients, Williams thought she was dealing with a new clinical entity. Because she was able to treat kwashiorkor by providing skim milk and other protein-rich foods, she viewed its cause as a deficiency of protein in diets that otherwise provided enough calories and other nutrients.[6]

Following World War II, nutrition surveys in Africa continued to identify kwashiorkor as the result of a "protein gap." The World Health Organization advocated the development of new protein sources from fish, soy, millet, or corn that could be used to prevent childhood malnutrition. In countries outside Africa, however, physicians were seeing a second form of childhood malnutrition, marasmus. They attributed this condition to deficiencies of calories *and* protein in children who were fed infant formula. In areas without clean water supplies, bottle-fed children, lacking the immunity provided by breast milk, readily acquired infectious diseases. Children with marasmus did not look swollen but instead appeared shriveled. But by the late 1950s the two conditions were considered different forms of the same starvation condition.

Young, growing children require protein and nutrients—as well as calories—in greater amounts for their size than do adults. Without adequate amounts of calories and the full range of required nutrients, they become ill much faster. Nutrition scientists in the 1970s realized that the emphasis on protein had been misplaced. Instead, the lack of protein was a symptom of diets containing too few calories as well as too few nutrients of all types.

When food intake was adequate in amount and variety, protein intake was also likely to be adequate, and the focus of international agencies shifted to the "energy gap." Without adequate calories, the body uses protein to meet its energy needs rather than to build new body tissues. With that understood, nutrition scientists began referring to chronic undernutrition in childhood as protein-calorie or protein-energy malnutrition.[7] Today even these terms have largely been replaced by others that refer to the specific effects of undernutrition: stunting, wasting, and underweight.

THE EFFECTS OF CHRONIC CALORIE DEPRIVATION

When measured against international growth standards, young children suffering from undernutrition are now most often described by these terms:

- *Stunted:* low height for age (chronic undernutrition)
- *Wasted:* low weight for height (acute undernutrition)
- *Underweight:* low weight for age (generalized undernutrition)

Stunting most often occurs in the first few months of life among children who are no longer breastfed and who suffer from chronically inadequate food, impaired immunity, and infectious disease. Wasting reflects more acute deprivation and the effects of chronic, repeated, or more severe infections. Underweight can be due to stunting, wasting, or both. The United Nations Children's Fund (UNICEF) says that one-third of children in the developing world are affected by stunting. Rates of the other conditions are lower, except in South Asia, where more than 40 percent of children are underweight and nearly 20 percent are wasted.[8] The extent of these conditions correlates closely with the number of calories available in the various regions.

Stunting, wasting, and underweight are not trivial problems. They contribute to some 3.5 million deaths per year and to 35 percent of childhood illnesses. They are responsible for more than 60 percent of childhood deaths from diarrhea, 50 percent from malaria and pneumonia, and 44 percent from measles. Unsurprisingly, the risk of death increases in proportion to the degree of food, nutrient, and calorie deprivation. Although some of these deaths are caused by vitamin and mineral deficiencies or inadequate breastfeeding, most are due to the combined effects of poor nutrition and infections.[9]

Nutritional deprivation also has long-lasting effects, such as poor performance in school and impaired cognitive function. Stunted children tend to have short stature as adults. Pregnant women of short stature face higher risks in childbirth, and they are more likely to produce underweight babies who continue the cycle of doing poorly in school, greater susceptibility to serious illness, and premature death.[10]

CLOSING THE CALORIE GAP

Over the years, international agencies have set goals for reducing the number of hungry people in the world. In 1996 the World Food Summit committed to cutting the number in half by 2015. The Millennium Development Goals set in 2000 by the United Nations call for a similar target and for monitoring progress through estimates of the proportion of underweight children and the percentage of people consuming minimal calories.[11]

How these goals are to be accomplished is a separate question. Numerous intervention studies have demonstrated the obvious: giving children enough food improves their growth, disease resistance, and survival. But feeding interventions, useful as they are, do not address the underlying causes of childhood malnutrition. Malnutrition results not only from lack of food but also from its causes: the political, social, and economic causes of poverty and

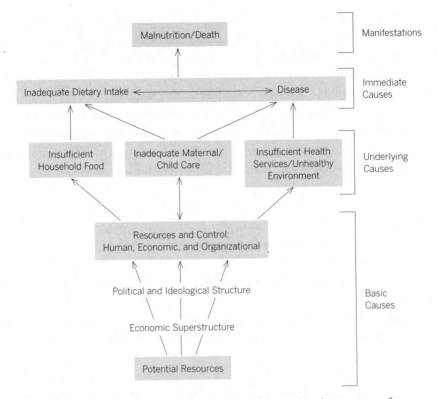

FIGURE 13. The complex political, social, and economic framework explaining causes of childhood malnutrition. Source: UNICEF, 1990 (see note 12).

its consequences, among them poor living conditions and inadequate access to safe water, sanitation, education, and medical care. UNICEF outlined this more comprehensive framework for understanding the causes of calorie deprivation in 1990, as shown in figure 13.[12]

The UNICEF conceptual framework distinguishes among immediate, underlying, and basic causes of malnutrition and death. Inadequate dietary intake and infectious disease are immediate causes of undernutrition. Interventions are critical at that level in the short term, but longer-term interventions do better when they address the underlying and basic causes of undernutrition. These inevitably have more to do with politics and economics than with food itself. Successful interventions focus on economic and social policies that promote adequate household food, maternal and child care, and health services. Such interventions also promote breastfeeding and the use of appropriate complementary foods (given as a supplement to breast milk) and dietary supplements, but they can be equally effective when focused on immunizations, sanitation measures, income support, and health care.[13] Any or all of these measures can improve the ability of children to learn and of adults to work and become more economically productive.

But acute malnutrition in a child is an emergency requiring immediate action. In recent years the treatment of severe wasting has been transformed by the use of high-calorie Ready-to-Use Therapeutic Food (RUTF), produced commercially. The most widely used RUTF is a sugar-sweetened, nutrient-fortified peanut butter packaged in 500-calorie portions. Children readily eat such products. With so many calories, it is not surprising that these foods reverse wasting and have proved to be effective in emergency situations.[14]

While the use of RUTFs may seem to solve the emergency nutrition problem, these products raise some troubling issues. They are expensive and divert resources from seeking more sustainable and affordable nutrient-dense foods produced by the local economy. In recent years the products have increasingly been proposed for use in nonemergency situations, and they provide an unwelcome opportunity for commercialization in the midst of humanitarian emergencies.[15]

Perhaps more important, emergency programs do not address the underlying causes of childhood malnutrition outlined in figure 13, especially the matter of income inequalities. When income disparities are reduced, rates of childhood malnutrition decline. Countries such as China, Thailand, and Brazil have reduced their poverty rates as a result of rapid economic growth. They also have invested in public health programs that provide safe water, education, immunizations, and access to health care. One gratifying result is that the prevalence of childhood stunting in Brazil dropped from 37 percent in 1974–75 to just 7 percent by 2006–07. China and Thailand reduced childhood malnutrition by half during that period.[16]

FOOD INSECURITY IN THE UNITED STATES

Anyone looking at Americans today would be hard-pressed to find many cases of childhood or adult stunting, wasting, or underweight. Such problems were readily observable in the late 1960s, however. Then, a CBS television documentary, *Hunger in America*, shocked the nation with its images of clearly undernourished children living in areas of deep poverty. Congress responded by expanding food assistance programs, and severe undernutrition disappeared from public view.[17]

Nutritional deficiencies may exist in the United States, but not because of food shortages. From the early 1900s to the early 1980s, the U.S. food supply provided an average of 3,200 calories a day per person. By the early 2000s the number had increased to 3,900 calories a day, and it has remained at that level ever since.[18] Some people, however, cannot afford to buy food. Americans are not necessarily starving, but many lack food security, a term defined by the USDA as a reliable ability to acquire sufficient food in socially acceptable ways.

The USDA divides food security into four ranges: high, marginal, low, and very low, depending on the degree to which a household lacks access to food. Only the category of very low food security is associated with typically disrupted eating patterns and reduced food intake. The USDA assesses the degree of food security among Americans through an annual survey of about 50,000 households. In 2010 it characterized 14.5 percent of U.S. households as food insecure, a percentage that translates to about 33 million adults and 16 million children, a shocking number unacceptable in so wealthy a country.

This percentage, unchanged from the previous year, maintained the highest levels recorded since the first such survey in 1995. It represented a sharp increase over the 11 percent recorded in 2008, most likely a result of deteriorating economic conditions and increased unemployment. Perhaps at the greatest risk of undernutrition are the 5 million or so children living in households with very low food security. This group constitutes the prime target of federal food assistance programs, a safety net under constant attack in an era of cost containment.[19]

CHAPTER 15

Could Restricting Calories Prolong Human Life?

Calorie deprivation, as we have seen, is difficult to endure and induces premature death in children and adults. Surely it should be avoided. But in 1935 Cornell professor Clive McCay and his colleagues noticed that when they fed diets deficient in nutrients to mice and rats, the animals grew more slowly. The researchers wondered whether the slowing down of early growth might affect how long the animals lived and decided to investigate that question. They established a feeding protocol for just-weaned male laboratory rat pups. For a few weeks they gave the baby rats in sequence:

- enough calories to survive but not enough to gain weight;
- a bit more food so the rats would gain some weight;
- just enough calories so the rats would maintain the new weight plateau but not gain more.

They repeated this feeding cycle throughout the lifetime of the animals.

As expected, the restricted rats gained weight, but in steps. But as the study continued, the investigators noticed something surprising. The intermittently starved rats lived nearly twice as long as their normally fed counterparts—an average of 820 days as compared to 483 days. Later the researchers observed similar effects in female rats.[1] Because both diets were carefully balanced in nutrients, the longer life span could have had only one cause: calorie restriction.

In subsequent years other investigators have done similar studies with similar results. These invariably show that calorie restriction—by 25 percent or more from normal intake levels—extends the life of rats and mice, as well as hamsters, rabbits, dogs, fish, flies, water fleas, worms, and yeast. For example, calorie restriction has been shown to extend the life of Labrador retrievers by an additional 14 months and to reduce their development of age-related diseases such as cancer and diabetes.[2]

No wonder calorie restriction is a major focus of current research on aging. These studies raise the intriguing possibility that calorie restriction might also extend human life.

CALORIE RESTRICTION: RHESUS MONKEYS

Before testing the idea on humans, it might be useful to find out if restricting calories extends the life of other primates. At least three separate studies are testing that hypothesis in rhesus monkeys. These studies require extraordinary commitments from researchers and funding agencies because rhesus monkeys live an average of twenty-seven years.

The first of these studies, conducted at the Wisconsin National Primate Research Center, began in 1989. The idea was to reduce the calorie intake of a group of monkeys by 30 percent and compare the health of that group to that of a matched control group of monkeys allowed to eat normally. The study originally included fifteen male monkeys in each group, all of them fully grown adults. In 1994 about as many more monkeys were added to the study population.

The investigators reported preliminary results in 2009. These were nothing short of sensational. Only 13 percent of the calorie-restricted monkeys had died of age-related causes by that time, as compared to 38 percent of the normally fed monkeys. The calorie-restricted monkeys weighed less, had lost most of their body fat, and displayed lower rates of diabetes, cancer, cardiovascular disease, and brain shrinkage compared to the controls.[3] But were the semistarved monkeys depressed, lethargic, obsessed with food, or less interested in sex, as was reported by participants in the Minnesota starvation study we discussed in chapter 13? The report said nothing about such matters.

Neither did reports from the other two studies. These have not gone on long enough to assess longevity. The National Institute on Aging is restricting calories in 120 monkeys. So far, it reports that the calorie-restricted animals weigh less and display reduced blood pressure and improved insulin sensitivity. The University of Maryland Primate Center has eight monkeys under calorie restriction and reports that this practice mitigates age-related disease. When asked to predict whether calorie restriction will increase longevity in rhesus monkeys, investigators at the National Institute on Aging said, "We think so."[4]

CALORIE RESTRICTION: HUMANS

Scientists are cautious about extrapolating findings in animals to humans, but the calorie-restriction analogy has some support. One line of evidence comes from observations of Japanese people living on the island of Okinawa. Dietary surveys in the 1960s and 1970s reported that adults in Okinawa consumed only 83 percent as many calories as the average person in Japan, and schoolchildren only 62 percent. The typical diet consisted of yellow root vegetables, sweet potatoes, green leafy vegetables, soybeans, and small amounts of meat and fish. The Okinawans were quite lean and maintained stable body weights well into their later years.

In 1995, life expectancy at birth for people on Okinawa was more than a year longer than for Japan as a whole—83.8 years compared to 82.3 (and 78.9 for the United States). But the difference later in life was even more impressive. At the age of 65, a woman could expect to live another 24.1 years and a man 18.5 years, a few years longer than their counterparts in well-fed areas. Mortality from cardiovascular disease and other age-related conditions was quite low in this population. Were these favorable statistics due to calorie restriction? The investigators said the health and longevity of these people might be due to classic advice given by Okinawan grandmothers: "Eat until you are 80 percent full."[5]

The Okinawa study is observational, and factors other than calorie restriction could have been responsible for the longer life spans. But at least one ongoing study is testing the effects of calorie restriction in humans. Funded by the National Institute on Aging, the study is titled "Comprehensive Assessment of Long-Term Effects of Reducing Intake of Energy," or CALERIE. The CALERIE study began preliminary pilot testing in 2002 at three centers: Tufts University, the Pennington Research Center in Louisiana, and Washington University in St. Louis.

The Pennington group reported results from the preliminary trial in 2007.

The pilot test divided participants into three groups of a dozen each. One group reduced calorie intake by 25 percent, another reduced it by 12.5 percent but increased energy expenditure by 12.5 percent, and a control group maintained usual calorie intake. After 24 weeks on these diets, the calorie-restricted and restricted-plus-exercise groups had lost about 10 percent of their initial body weights and 24 percent of their body fat in comparison to the control group.[6] The participants in both calorie-restricted groups had lower body core temperatures and lower fasting insulin levels than those in the control group. Based on the rodent and monkey studies, these measures appear to be biomarkers for increased longevity.[7] Like the men in the Minnesota study, the calorie-restricted subjects also had lower basal energy expenditures.

With these preliminary results in hand, investigators launched the full CALERIE study in 2007. This involved the same three sites but a much larger group of 250 volunteers, ages 25 to 45 years. CALERIE simplified the protocol and assigned the volunteers to one of just two groups: calorie restriction by 25 percent or a normal diet. The study period was to last only two years.[8]

In some respects, CALERIE duplicated the Minnesota semistarvation experiments, but it was less extreme. The study was not expected to determine whether calorie restriction extends life. Instead, its purpose was to provide information about the safety and feasibility of reduced calorie intake for humans and whether the effects of calorie restriction on chronic disease risk factors in humans might be similar to those found in rhesus monkeys.

In 2009 a reporter, Jon Gertner, interviewed participants in the CALERIE study for an article in the *New York Times Magazine*. Most had lost about 15 percent of their body weight in the first year and adapted to an intake of calories that supported their new weight. They told Gertner that they felt hungry for the first few weeks of the study but eventually got used to eating less. What about their mental health? They attended individual and group counseling sessions once or twice a week to help them comply with the low-calorie regimen.[9] If nothing else, the study proved that it is possible to find people who are willing to comply with calorie-restricted diets under peacetime conditions.

The CALERIE volunteers reported much less misery than the conscientious objectors participating in the Minnesota study, no doubt because CALERIE was much less restrictive. Once the volunteers lost weight, their calorie needs were less. They were also free to live their usual lives. In contrast, the Minnesota study participants were required to eat all their meals on-site, and their calorie allotment was progressively reduced over the course of the study to force a 25 percent weight loss.[10] At the time of this writing, the results of this study had not been published. We look forward to seeing them.

VOLUNTARY CALORIE RESTRICTION

The early experimental evidence that calorie deprivation extends the life span of animals was enough to convince a group of dedicated individuals to choose calorie restriction as a lifestyle. In 1994 they formed the Calorie Restriction Society to attract other members who might be "interested in learning and practicing the genuine life-extending principles of Calorie Restriction." The society's website home page displays a graph of the effects of calorie restriction on life extension in mice. We reproduce it in figure 14.[11]

The society suggests that its members will achieve longer and healthier lives by taking in fewer calories from food and making up for potential nutrient deficiencies with supplements. Although the society does not recommend a specific level of calorie restriction, it suggests a weight loss of 15 to 25 percent as a reasonable target. The society provides extensive advice to its members about how to achieve this loss while still meeting nutrient needs.

As you might imagine, researchers cannot wait to study practitioners of calorie restriction. Scientists at Washington University in St. Louis recruited 18 of them for studies of cardiovascular risk factors. Some volunteers had been restricting calories for an average of six years and a few for as many as fifteen years. The investigators compared the volunteers' risk factors for age-related disease to those of a comparable control group eating an unrestricted diet. Society members were about 20 percent leaner than the comparison group and exhibited much lower levels of blood cholesterol, blood pressure, and indicators of inflammation.[12] Similar studies of calorie restrictors are now under way at the University of California School of Medicine in San Francisco (UCSF).[13]

The Calorie Restriction Society is quite clear about the difficulties involved in following its practices. It recognizes the considerable discomfort of self-starvation and tells members that they are likely to experience hunger, cold, and changes in appearance. Women will experience menstrual irregularities. Testosterone levels will decrease in men. Practitioners will obsess about food, upset their families, and make friends uncomfortable at social

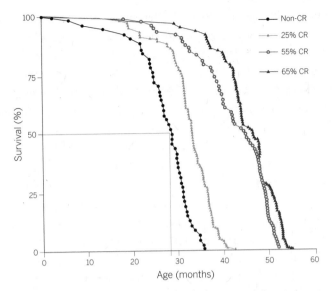

FIGURE 14. Mice fed calorie-restricted (CR) diets survive longer than normally fed (non-CR) animals. The graph appears on the Calorie Restriction Society website at www.crsociety.org. It is rather freely adapted from a 1986 study in which mice were fed diets that differed in vitamin, mineral, and protein content as well as degree of calorie restriction, making it difficult to know whether similar results would be obtained with mice fed diets of higher nutritional quality (see note 11).

events. For the members of the society, whatever it takes to achieve semistarvation must seem worth the benefits.

But what are the benefits? It is not at all certain that this level of calorie restriction will extend human life. Despite much searching, we cannot find evidence that people who experienced starvation at any time during their lives live longer than those who did not. If anything, very early starvation is associated with an increase in risk factors for chronic disease later in life.[14] People with anorexia nervosa do not necessarily live longer than their better-fed counterparts. Extreme calorie restriction is demonstrably life threatening. Milder semistarvation—even with nutritional supplements—seems unlikely to promote long-term physical or mental health in human populations. Most compelling, large-scale studies of the relationship of body weight to mortality invariably find notably higher death rates among people whose body weights are below ranges considered normal.[15]

Without evidence to support the benefits of calorie restriction, expert opinions on this practice vary all over the place. In 2006 *Biogerontology* reported the opinions of twelve experts on human aging. Five felt that calorie restriction can extend human longevity, six said it cannot, and one said it was too early to decide. Still others believe that calorie restriction might extend life spans but not by much, mainly because humans live longer than rats and mice. And some say that avoiding obesity ought to extend longevity by three to thirteen years. But statisticians repeatedly find that body weights within ranges considered normal are associated with the lowest mortality rates.[16]

Researchers at the National Institute on Aging say we will never know for sure whether calorie restriction promotes longevity, because a definitive human study would have to last one hundred years or more. Instead, they have begun to look at drug approaches to life extension. They are studying the use of "calorie restriction mimetics" such as antioxidants and resveratrol (the chemical in red grapes that is more concentrated in red wines). If these chemicals work, they might delay the onset of age-related diseases without requiring people to change their diets. Unfortunately, nothing in nutrition has ever been that easy, and the results of these studies have not shown much promise to date.[17]

In looking at the research on calorie restriction, we are impressed by the strong and consistent evidence for its ability to reduce risk factors for heart disease, stroke, type 2 diabetes, and some cancers. If nothing else, the calorie restriction studies confirm the substantial health benefits of avoiding overweight and obesity. Calorie control strategies could translate into more years of healthy life regardless of their effect on longevity.

At the moment, scientists have not been able to determine the degree to which calories must be restricted to achieve these benefits or the stage of life at which restriction would be most effective. But surely reductions of 25 percent are neither necessary nor desirable. Hunger is not a pleasant sensation, and the social delights of eating and sharing meals are deeply ingrained aspects of human culture. Is adding a year or two of life worth an entire lifetime of semistarvation and struggle to overcome basic physiological drives to eat? Members of the Calorie Restriction Society may think so, but we enjoy the pleasures of the table too much to agree.

PART FIVE

Too Many Calories

In the next chapters we address questions about what happens when you eat more calories than you expend, put on weight, become overweight or obese, and then try to take the weight off. Overweight and obesity are now *global* phenomena. In many countries the numbers of obese people exceed the numbers who are undernourished and hungry. The importance of obesity as a worldwide public health problem has encouraged researchers to investigate trends and their causes and determine the levels of overweight and obesity that increase health risks. In our attempt here to define the number of excess calories that must be eaten to gain weight, and to explain why some people seem to put on weight more easily than others, we find ourselves confronted by a research literature of oceanic proportions, a good deal of it contradictory and much of it exceedingly difficult to interpret.

Weight-loss studies typically require people to vary either the number of calories they consume or the proportions of carbohydrate, fat, and protein in their diets. But it is impossible to vary one dietary component without changing the proportions of others as well. Unless conducted on people isolated in metabolic wards, such studies necessarily involve "free-living" volunteers—people who go about their daily lives doing whatever else they usually do while supposedly following the prescribed diets. Adherence to experimental diets is not always easy in this situation. To determine adherence, investigators must depend on self-reports of food consumption. These, alas, are notoriously unreliable (see chapter 10). Although investigators may measure changes in weight and related risk factors (blood pressure, blood cholesterol, blood glucose, insulin), they can never be sure whether what they are measuring is due to the diet or to some other behavior or characteristic of free-living people.

Because dieting is strongly countered by basic biological drives to eat, the duration of the studies is another concern. Many studies show impressive weight loss within the first six months. But if the studies last longer, participants tend to regain much or all of the weight. And the longer a study continues, the greater the chance that its subjects will stop participating and become lost to follow-up. Studies with high dropout rates—and this, it turns out, includes virtually all long-term weight-loss trials—require especially careful interpretation. Individuals who stick to trial protocols may not be typical of the group as a whole. Other researchers attempting to make sense of this messy research situation may well interpret the studies differently and come to different conclusions, but in this part of the book we have been especially cautious in our interpretations in order to provide the best reading we can of the current evidence.

Dieting, we repeat, comes up against physiological defenses against weight loss. It is not impossible to overcome these defenses and lose or maintain weight. But it is not easy, especially in the context of a food environment constructed to entice you to eat more at every opportunity. Many popular books and programs propose simplifying dieting by restricting one or another source of calories. They insist that diets low in fat or, conversely, carbohydrate will help you lose weight. But does the source of calories really make a difference? To address that question, we look at real-world studies that have attempted to find out whether dieters do better on one kind of diet or another. Obesity, these studies show, is another one of those complex biological problems with multiple causes and no simple solution. Do calories count? We think so, but read on.

CHAPTER 16

An Introduction to Obesity

If you habitually eat more calories than you expend, you will gain weight, and most of that weight will be in the form of fat. A pound of body fat tissue contains about 3,500 calories. You can work this out using the Atwater Value: 9 calories per gram times 454 grams per pound. Even without a calculator, it should be obvious that this sum comes to more than 3,500 calories. But fat tissue contains only about 85 percent fat; the rest is water, protein, and other such things. Multiplying 4 times 454 by 0.85 gives you a number that conveniently rounds off to 3,500. As with all numbers referring to calories, this figure is approximate and varies among individuals. And because calories are not deposited into fat tissue with 100 percent efficiency, you need to overeat more than 3,500 calories to add a pound of body fat. But whatever the exact count, you will gain weight in proportion to the amount your calorie intake exceeds the number you expend.

THE BODY MASS INDEX (BMI)

The world is awash in overeating. Substantial percentages of the population of most countries—all but the very poorest—are considered overweight or obese. Such percentages are usually based on the body mass index (BMI), a single number that summarizes the relationship of body weight to height. Computing a BMI involves another of those nonintuitive formulas. Try this:

BMI equals weight in kilograms divided by height in meters squared.

TABLE 19   BODY MASS INDEX (BMI) ADULT
WEIGHT-FOR-HEIGHT CLASSIFICATIONS

Classification	BMI
Underweight	<18.5
Normal weight	18.5–24.9
Overweight	25.0–29.9
Obese	>30
Extremely obese	>40

Translating the formula into pounds and inches helps only a little:

BMI equals weight in pounds times 703 divided by
height in inches times itself.

The Centers for Disease Control and Prevention (CDC) solves the calculation problem by providing handy online BMI calculators for adults and children.[1] The BMI provides a convenient, if not always accurate, way to categorize people of varying weights for their height. For example, a woman who weighs 130 pounds and is 5 feet 6 inches tall has a BMI of 21. Table 19 shows what that number means for an adult.

The BMI classification system works fairly well as an indicator of body fat content, which otherwise can be measured with reasonable accuracy only by methods that tend to be complicated, indirect, inconvenient, and expensive.[2] Given that the BMI is a continuous variable—it can fall anywhere along the full spectrum of heights and weights—its cutoff points are arbitrary. The BMI penalizes people with relatively high muscle and bone mass, which do not carry the same metabolic risks as body fat. But by and large the BMI is a useful—a good enough—starting point for evaluating the health risks of excessive calorie intake and its consequences. These risks increase slowly but continuously with increases in BMI above the range considered normal and increase sharply in the higher BMI ranges.[3]

THE HEALTH RISKS OF OBESITY

Concerns about obesity would not be so pronounced if this condition were simply a matter of appearance. Excessive calorie intake does not always cause disease, but when it does the problems can be serious. And the list of such problems is long, including such leading causes of death and disability as coronary heart disease, high blood pressure, type 2 diabetes, certain cancers (endometrial, breast, colon), stroke, liver and gallbladder disease, sleep apnea and respiratory problems, osteoarthritis, and gynecological problems such as abnormal menses and infertility.[4]

The probability of developing these conditions, while nowhere near 100 percent, increases with increasing overweight, as does the probability of developing several of them simultaneously. The combination of such symptoms as high blood pressure, high blood triglycerides (fat), high blood sugar, and excess fat in the abdomen has its own name: the metabolic syndrome. Obesity and its consequences affect quality of life and may lead to premature mortality. Compounding these personal costs for individuals are the societal costs of medical care and lost productivity, estimated at hundreds of billions of dollars annually in the United States alone.[5]

Many of the metabolic abnormalities that result from obesity can be corrected by rather modest weight losses. The American Heart Association; the National Heart, Lung and Blood Institute; and the American Diabetes Association advise a gradual 7 to 10 percent reduction in body weight over a period of six to twelve months—meaning 21 to 30 pounds for someone weighing 300 pounds. To accomplish this loss, they advise a diet that reduces calories, minimizes high-calorie, highly processed foods of low nutritional value ("junk" foods), and emphasizes fruits, vegetables, and whole grains. They also advise 30 minutes a day of moderate-to-intense physical activity. This is standard dietary advice for everyone, dieting or not, and consistent with U.S. Dietary Guidelines.[6] In theory, this advice should be easy to follow. In practice, as we explain in later chapters, for many people it is anything but.

TRENDS IN ADULT OBESITY: UNITED STATES

For many years the percentage of the U.S. population considered overweight or obese stayed about the same. Surveys from the early 1960s until the late 1970s identified about 32 percent of the population as overweight and a bit more than 13 percent as obese. After that, percentages of obesity (but not overweight) rose sharply—from about 15 percent in the 1976–80 survey to 23 percent in the survey of 1988–94. By 2007–08, 34 percent of the adult population had reached a BMI in the range considered obese. When people in the overweight and obese BMI ranges were considered together, the total constituted an astonishing 68 percent of the U.S. population: 64 percent of women and 72 percent of men. Even higher percentages were observed among members of minority groups. And from 1988–94 to 2005–06, the percentage of extremely obese, those with a BMI greater than 40, doubled from about 3 percent to 6 percent.[7]

Another way to look at these trends is to look at changes in average body size—the heights and weights of the population. From the early 1960s to the early 2000s, men and women gained an average of about 20 pounds, but height increased by only about 1 inch. Men went from 174 to 195 pounds and women from 145 to 165 pounds.[8] These are *average* weight gains. Some people did not gain weight at all over this period, while many others gained a good deal more than 20 pounds.

If 68 percent of a population is overweight or obese and worldwide trends are headed in the same direction, you can understand why obesity is considered epidemic. Although government surveys show some slowing down of the rise in obesity, predictions of future trends tend to be dire. A group at Harvard, for example, observes that people are more likely to be obese if their friends are obese, suggesting that obesity, like other epidemic diseases, is "contagious." If everyone around you is overweight, then overweight becomes the new normal. The pessimistic Harvard group thinks that rates of obesity (though not necessarily overweight) will continue to rise and eventually level off at about 42 percent. But even this prediction seems modest to international experts who believe rates will reach 50 percent by 2030, causing catastrophic increases in the health and economic burdens of governments throughout the world.[9]

What is particularly distressing about obesity statistics is that similar trends apply to children. The CDC has developed BMI standards for children based on national surveys of child growth over the past fifty years. For children ages 2 to 19, overweight is defined as a BMI of greater than the 85th percentile for age but less than the 95th percentile. Children with a BMI in the 85th percentile are heavier for their heights than 85 percent of other children of the same age. Children are considered obese when their weight-for-height measurement exceeds the 95th percentile for their age.[10]

The trends alarm public health officials. The percentage of obese children doubled and in some age groups tripled from 1976–80 to 2007–08. During this period the percent of children ages 2 to 5 defined as obese doubled from 5 to 10 percent. Among children ages 6 to 11 rates of obesity nearly tripled from 7 to 20 percent, and among children ages 12 to 19 it more than tripled, from

5 to 18 percent. Among children in minority population groups, the percentages are even higher.[11]

OBESITY TRENDS: INTERNATIONAL

The population of the United States is not alone in storing more calories than it needs. In parts of Europe, the Middle East, and Latin America, more than 60 percent of adults over the age of 15 are overweight or obese. England, Greece, and Germany, for example, report rates only slightly lower than those in the United States. Worldwide, nearly 10 percent of men and 14 percent of women were estimated to be obese in 2008. These percentages represent a doubling since 1980. Even in countries where significant undernutrition still exists, percentages of overweight and obese people are rising. In 2008, public health officials estimated that nearly 1.5 billion adults in the world were overweight, among them 500 million who were obese.[12] For the first time in world history, the number of overweight people meets or exceeds the number of people defined as undernourished. While this should sound like wonderful economic progress, it threatens to drain the economies of countries that can ill afford a workforce with high levels of disability or the attendant costs of treating obesity-related chronic diseases.

Taken together, the statistics indicate that people who have enough money are piling on the calories, in a trend that has accelerated since the 1980s. In chapter 21 we discuss what happened in the early 1980s to initiate such trends, but much evidence leads us and others to conclude that many aspects of the current environment of food overabundance "conspire" to override physiological controls of energy balance. But before getting to that, let's take a look at how many excess calories it takes to override those controls and cause you to gain weight, and how many fewer you have to eat to lose whatever weight you gained.

CHAPTER 17

Calories and Weight Gain
Another Complex Relationship

Increases in body weight are easier to measure than increases in body fat, but excessive body fat is the cause of metabolic problems. If you eat too many calories for the number you expend, most of them will end up as body fat. Fatty tissue is an ideal place to store calories, not least because its capacity seems unlimited in some people. Very obese people can accumulate very large amounts of body fat, and magazines delight in publishing articles about people who weigh 1,000 pounds or more.[1]

What complicates discussions of body fat is that it is good to have some, just not too much. Fat insulates and has survival value. The storage of calories in body fat explains why extremely obese people are able to survive fasting for periods of a year or more, whereas the Irish hunger strikers we discussed in chapter 13 lasted only two months.[2] The fat content of individuals can and does vary widely. An elite athlete might be 5 percent body fat, while someone who is obese might be more than 50 percent fat. On average, women carry more body fat than men, 25 percent as compared to 18 percent. A man who weighs 150 pounds could easily be carrying 27 pounds of pure fat sequestered in fatty tissue. This amount represents a storage capacity of more than 110,000 calories (27 pounds × 454 grams per pound × 9 calories per gram).

The body stores fat in specialized cells (adipocytes) that collectively make up fatty (adipose) tissue. As more fat is stored, the cells increase in size and distribution. In some people, the cells also increase in number. You can see what fatty tissues look like when you trim the fat from a steak or pork chop. The fat is dense and white or yellow. You have fat like this under your skin, where it insulates. Much more fat is distributed in the upper and lower body and belly. Like all living tissues, fatty tissue is suffused with blood vessels and other fluids and is not really solid.[3] This explains why its calorie content is about 3,500 per pound rather than the 4,100 that would be expected from multiplying 9 calories per gram by 454 grams per pound.

When you eat an enormous mixed meal containing loads of calories from proteins, fats, and carbohydrates, your body preferentially metabolizes the carbohydrates to produce energy and store glycogen. Any remaining carbohydrates are converted to fat and stored in fatty tissue. This metabolic preference is precisely the rationale behind the New York City Health Department's "Are you pouring on the pounds?" campaign in 2011.[4] The department wanted New Yorkers to understand that sugary soft drinks can make people fat, just as eating fat can.

The body's use of carbohydrates depends on calories. When two conditions are met—the diet contains enough calories to meet energy needs *and* enough carbohydrate to maintain blood glucose levels—the body uses hardly any fat to produce energy. Absorbed fatty acids go right into body fat. In contrast, when the diet contains too few calories to meet energy needs, the body uses all the available carbohydrates to fuel the brain. In that situation, fat stores break down to fatty acids, which the body uses to supply most of its energy needs, as we explained in chapter 13.

OVERFEEDING BY LARGE AMOUNTS

Scientists have long been interested in what happens to calorie balance during weight loss and gain. Just as Ancel Keys studied weight loss under conditions of near starvation, more recently investigators have induced volunteers to stuff themselves and gain weight. Ethan Sims, for example, did some early studies of experimental obesity at the University of Vermont.[5] In the 1960s, when such studies were still permitted, Sims and his colleagues got eight "volunteers"—in quotation marks because they were incarcerated at the Vermont state prison—to gorge themselves until they increased their body weights by 25 percent.

Sims's studies did not measure calorie intake or expenditure. They were conducted before the use of doubly labeled water techniques became common, and the way they presented the results makes it hard to know exactly how many calories the volunteers were overeating. From our reading of the studies, we guess that the prisoners increased their intake by 3,500 to 4,000 calories per day over and above their usual intake, and some consumed as many as 10,000 calories a day.

After six months or so the men succeeded in increasing their body weights by 18 to 31 percent, most of it as body fat. At that point they were allowed to eat whatever they wanted and were placed on a vigorous exercise program. Eventually their body weights returned to previous levels. Sims reported that the men who had gained the extra weight most rapidly were the ones who took the longest to get it off by the end of the study. Using the methods then available, Sims was unable to account for all the energy consumed by the prisoners—not all of the excess calories went into fat—and he speculated that they might have increased spontaneous physical activity or generated more energy as heat.

Such experiments are no longer permitted under federal ethical guidelines, and we are not aware of any others examining this question using incarcerated prisoners. We discuss some overfeeding experiments with free-living volunteers in the next chapter. Whatever the results of those experiments, a natural experiment is now in progress in which people all over the world are gaining weight. Observers of this trend are intensely curious about the number of excess calories that it takes to cause people to gain weight. Researchers have addressed this problem by estimating the size of the reduction in calorie intake needed either to prevent weight gain or to reverse the gain in weight that has already occurred.

PREVENTING FURTHER WEIGHT GAIN: SMALL CHANGES

Sims's studies involved overeating by several thousand calories a day. It is easy to understand why anyone would gain weight doing that. But what if you overeat by a much smaller amount? We cannot count the number of times we have heard people say that if you eat one extra Oreo cookie a day— 50 calories—you will gain 5 pounds in a year. This notion comes from a theoretical calculation: 50 calories a day times 365 days a year, divided by 3,500 calories per pound, equals 5 pounds of fat.

James Hill and his colleagues at the University of Colorado looked at the same CDC data on obesity trends that we summarized in the previous chapter. They compared average body weights reported in the CDC surveys of 1988–94 to those reported in 1999–2000. From this comparison they estimated that adults (ages 20 to 40) gained an average of about 2 pounds per year and that 90 percent of this group had gained less than 5 pounds a year.[6] This estimation assumed that the study subjects did not change energy expenditure over that time.

From the theoretical calculation, the Hill group assumed that a 5-pound weight gain would require the storage of only 50 calories a day as body fat. People who gained less than 5 pounds must have been depositing fewer than 50 calories a day. The researchers made one more assumption: calories are deposited in body fat at about 50 percent efficiency. Therefore, gaining 5 pounds in the course of a year requires an average intake of 100 excess calories per day.

If this is true, it means that to prevent that 5-pound weight gain, people would have had to decrease the calories they were consuming by 100 per day, increase energy expenditure by that amount, or make 50-calorie changes in both. According to Hill, a shift like this could easily be accomplished by small changes that would require nothing more than consuming one less sugary soft drink a day or walking an additional 2,000 steps (one mile). Hill's analysis suggests that these small changes are just what it will take to prevent current rates of obesity from rising further.

Hill and his colleague Dr. John Peters established a foundation called America on the Move to promote this approach. The "small steps" idea has enormous popular appeal, especially among government agencies. The USDA's National Institute of Food and Agriculture, for example, developed a partnership with America on the Move to promote the concept of taking 2,000 more steps or eating 100 fewer calories each day.[7]

In a study of overweight children, researchers at the Baylor College of Medicine applied an analytical method similar to Hill's to estimate what it would take to prevent children from becoming overweight. Their studies found that overweight children gain weight much more rapidly than adults and store an estimated 144 excess calories a day rather than 50 or 100. Assuming that those calories were deposited at 50 percent efficiency, the Baylor group suggested that overweight children would need to reduce their energy intake by nearly 300 calories per day to prevent further weight gain. Those who were putting weight on more quickly would need to reduce energy intake by as much as 500 calories a day to stay at their current weights.[8] Changes of this size are anything but small.

BUT WHAT WOULD IT TAKE TO REVERSE OBESITY?

Most people unconsciously adjust calorie intake and expenditure over time so as to maintain stable weights for years. This should not be difficult to do within a range of 100 calories. The problem is that once you gain weight, you have to eat more calories to maintain it. Larger bodies have higher basal metabolic rates and expend more calories in physical activity. They "demand" that you eat more calories than you did when you weighed less.

An example may help clarify this point. Suppose that a 150-pound man overeats calories over time and puts on an additional 6 pounds. For someone of his initial weight, the 6-pound gain adds about 65 calories a day to his total energy requirement. To return to 150 pounds, he would have to reduce his current level of energy intake by at least 65 calories per day. But if he is continuing to gain weight, he must be eating his original number of calories, plus the extra 65, plus the additional calories needed to produce any new weight increase. Eventually his weight may equilibrate at a new "settling point" that requires the higher calorie intake to maintain. If you are constantly gaining weight, you must be constantly eating more calories than you need.

Sometimes people who are gaining weight are eating many more calories than they need. According to measurements of energy expenditure reviewed by the Institute of Medicine, a man weighing 150 pounds whose weight rises to 210 pounds over time will require an additional 400 calories a day to maintain the new weight.[9] If this man wants to return to 150 pounds he must reduce his habitual intake by 400 calories a day plus whatever calorie increments caused him to gain weight in the first place. This is why we think it is a good idea to monitor weight gain carefully. You only need to restrict calories by a small amount to reduce a moderate weight gain, but reversing a larger gain requires much more severe calorie restriction.

Researchers at the National Institutes of Health have developed mathematical models to estimate the kinds of changes in calorie intake that would be needed to maintain a reduced body weight in people who used to be obese. Their models suggest, for example, that if a 176-pound woman managed to get down to 140 pounds, she would have to reduce her intake by 300 calories a day to maintain the new weight, and do so permanently. Another group of obesity researchers used a similar model to predict that returning the body weights of the U.S. population to levels typical of 1980 would require Americans to eat 380 fewer calories a day on average than are presently consumed.[10]

Boyd Swinburn and his colleagues at Deakin University in Australia have also tackled this problem by using the same U.S. survey data, in this case from 1971–76 to 1999–2000. As a basis for comparison, they drew on the USDA's data on food availability—the number of calories available in the food supply, adjusted for spoilage and other losses (see chapter 10). During that period, the number of available calories in the food supply increased by 300 for children and 500 for adults, amounts the researchers judge more than sufficient to explain the observed weight gains. To reverse obesity trends and return to body weights observed in the 1970s, children would have to reduce their daily calorie intakes by the equivalent of one large soda and a small French fries. Adults would have to eliminate the calorie equivalent of one large hamburger or increase physical activity by hundreds of calories a day. An online interactive Body Weight Simulator permits individuals to calculate the size of their own energy gap and is entertaining as well as instructive.[11]

In a review of the "how many calories would it take" question, researchers Martijn Katan and David Ludwig examined the same evidence used by other investigators but also included mathematical models that predict the effects of changes in energy intake on body weight. By their calculations, a 25-year-old person with a BMI of 25 (the top of the normal range) would have to increase energy intake, decrease physical activity, or both by nearly 700 calories a day to reach a BMI of 35 and become obese by age 50. For adolescents, the energy gap that leads to extremes of obesity is even higher. Impossibly high as an excess of 700 calories a day may seem, several pediatricians have told us that they frequently see obese children in their practices who admit to consuming 1,000 to 2,000 calories a day from soft drinks alone. Some studies provide research support for numbers that high, especially among obese adolescents.[12]

These kinds of investigations make a strong case for the idea that the level of calorie excess that causes and maintains weight gain for many people, especially obese children, is more than 100 calories per day and sometimes much more. Reversing this level of calorie imbalance will be difficult for most people to manage. They cannot do it alone. As Katan and Ludwig suggest, "Rather, an effective public health approach to obesity prevention will require fundamental changes in the food supply and the social infrastructure. Changes of this nature depend on more stringent regulation of the food industry, agricultural policy informed by public health, and investments by government in the social environment to promote physical activity."

We think so too.

Do Excess Calories Make Some People Gain Weight Faster than Others?

Everyone knows people who are not especially athletic but seem to be able to eat anything in front of them and never gain an ounce. Are they not telling the truth about what they eat? Or do they really burn off calories more efficiently than everyone else? Some people seem to be able to lose weight effortlessly, while for others it is an interminable struggle. Here we take up the matter of individual variation in response to excessive calorie intake.

The overfeeding studies described in the previous chapter answer this question to some extent. In response to eating thousands of extra calories a day, all of the Vermont prisoners put on weight, but some gained more weight than others, and they gained it faster. Other studies have confirmed that observation.

Investigators at the Mayo Clinic, for example, gave 16 men an extra 1,000 calories a day for 8 weeks. The men gained an average of 10 pounds, but some gained as few as 3 or as many as 16. Genetics has something to do with such variation. When investigators fed 1,000 excess calories a day to pairs of identical twins for nearly three months, the twins gained nearly 18 pounds on average, but the range was 10 to 30 pounds. Genetics seemed to be the critical factor because the variation in weight gain between the two members of any one pair of twins was much smaller than the variation in weight gain between one pair of twins and any other pair.[1]

RESPONSE TO CALORIE EXCESS

We know people who deliberately go to gyms to work off excess calories. Beyond such exemplary behavior, researchers suggest three ways in which innate individual differences in physiology might affect responses to over-feeding: thermic effects of food, brown fat, and spontaneous physical activity (fidgeting).

Thermic Effects of Food

Eating, as we explained in chapter 7, induces a measurable rise in heat production. Perhaps some people burn off more of the extra calories as heat? Although this idea sounds promising, research to date suggests that thermic effects are unlikely to be a major way to get rid of excess energy. Instead, studies conclude that heat losses from thermic effects increase in proportion to the number of calories in a meal. Just as larger bodies produce more heat, so do larger meals. And when people eat too much, they gain weight—mainly body fat—in proportion to the number of excess calories consumed. Larger bodies take more calories to maintain and move, but meal size is the critical factor. Large and small people who eat meals of the same nutrient composition and number of calories lose the same amount of heat from thermic effects.[2]

Brown Fat

In the 1970s, scientists interested in weight and obesity were fascinated to discover that the bodies of normal-weight mice and rats have a darker-colored, highly metabolically active fat tissue, which they called brown fat. In rodents this fat seemed to be involved in regulating body temperature. When the animals got cold, the brown fat cells produced more heat to maintain body temperature. This was an interesting observation, but what really excited the investigators was their discovery that letting rats and mice eat their choice of a variety of junk foods high in calories seemed to ratchet up the metabolism of brown fat so that the extra calories burned off. They were even more excited to identify drugs that stimulated the metabolism of brown fat in rats and mice.[3]

These were thrilling discoveries. If brown fat worked the same way in humans, changing the diet or finding the right drug could solve the obesity problem just like that. For a few years brown fat seemed to be *the* most promising avenue for obesity research. But subsequent research proved disappointing. Brown fat is indeed present in humans, especially infants, but its amounts start to decline soon after birth. Worse, the drugs that stimulated the metabolism of brown fat in rodents did not work in humans. For twenty years or so, we did not hear much about brown fat and human calorie regulation.

But interest in brown fat is now experiencing a revival. Recent studies show that humans do have detectable amounts of brown fat and that it responds to cold exposure in much the same way as in rodents. However, brown fat does not seem to respond to cold as efficiently in obese men as in lean men, perhaps because extra body fat insulates against the cold.[4] Still, these observations are sending researchers off again to look for drugs that might stimulate brown fat metabolism. Skeptics urge caution. Being cold is an uncomfortable way to use extra calories and might induce hunger and overeating. Brown fat remains under active investigation, and we expect to hear more about it in the years ahead.

Fidgeting

Could individual variations in rates of spontaneous physical activity be responsible for variations in weight gain during overfeeding? The Mayo Clinic investigators addressed this very question in their study. They carried out doubly labeled water experiments to measure the total energy expenditure of their overfed volunteers. The investigators also measured the volunteers' basal metabolic rates (BMRs) and energy expenditures during prescribed activities. The results? Neither the BMRs nor prescribed activity levels could explain the observed differences in fat deposition among their volunteers. Instead, the Mayo Clinic researchers concluded that the differences in fat deposition must have been due to what they called non-exercise activity thermogenesis, abbreviated NEAT and known commonly as fidgeting.[5]

NEAT, the investigators explained, includes thumb twiddling, standing as opposed to sitting or lying down, and other kinds of nervous twitching. They measured the calorie contribution of NEAT activities before and during the overeating trial. The change was remarkable. On average, the overeating volunteers increased their NEAT expenditure by 330 calories per day. But the range, as is so often the case, was substantial. At the extremes, one volunteer reduced NEAT activities by 100 calories a day, but another increased it by 690 calories. Most impressive, the volunteers whose NEAT expenditures increased the most during the overeating phase deposited the least amount of body fat.

If you think it might be difficult to assess levels of spontaneous physical activity, you would be right. In an attempt to do this, investigators at the

National Institutes of Health had the bright idea of using radar to monitor every movement of volunteers housed in a room-size respiratory calorimeter for 24 hours. They ended up convincing 177 people to participate in such experiments. Among these individuals, spontaneous physical activity accounted for calorie expenditures that varied from 100 to 800 calories per day.[6]

Neuroscientists are just beginning to understand how NEAT might be regulated. The brain is involved, as are some of the same signals that regulate food intake (see chapter 12), indicating that physiological controls of spontaneous physical activity may be another way the body regulates energy balance.[7] One attractive area of investigation is the extent to which voluntary physical activities might influence involuntary spontaneous activity.

The word *fidgeting* has negative connotations, as the behavior can be irritating to watch. Obesity researchers note that adults often try to restrain children from their natural fidgeting behavior by telling kids to be quiet, sit still, or "stop that" and diagnosing them with behavioral issues. Some researchers prefer to view fidgeting as a natural biological behavior that deserves encouragement as a way to increase physical activity and prevent obesity. Preliminary results of a small study suggest that giving school kids desks that allow them to stand while working causes them to expend more calories and, as a bonus, to improve their behavior and classroom performance.[8] Think about that the next time your kid's wiggling drives you nuts.

As we've seen, the number of calories expended in spontaneous movement can be large enough to account for individual variations in weight gain during overeating. This idea suggests simple strategies for adding to calorie expenditure. Whenever possible, stand rather than sit. Stand while using a computer or reading. Spend less time watching television. Pace the back of the room while attending long meetings. If people seem distracted by your behavior, you can simply explain that fidgeting is part of your weight-maintenance program.

RESPONSE TO DIETING

On the intake side of calorie balance, a typical response to weight gain is to go on a diet. Dieting has major economic implications, as it has spawned entire industries devoted to selling advice, weight loss products, books, and drug and surgical therapies. In 2009 the value of the diet industries in the United

States was estimated at nearly $60 billion, but this figure pales against the total cost of obesity to individuals and society.[9]

That the average American wants to lose weight is a given. A national survey of 185,000 people found substantial percentages who said they were dieting even though their weights were within ranges considered normal: 10 percent of men and 29 percent of women. The percentages were much higher among individuals who were overweight (36 percent of men, 60 percent of women) and obese (63 percent of men, 70 percent of women). Half of the people trying to lose weight said they were doing so by eating fewer calories, but only about 20 percent claimed to be exercising as well.[10]

Reducing calorie intake is famously difficult. For one thing, it is not fun. For another, metabolism slows down in proportion to weight loss. Once you lose weight, you need to eat fewer calories to maintain your reduced weight. And you cannot go back to the old habits that made you gain weight in the first place. If you are trying to restrict calories, you are confronting your basic biological drive to eat and to defend against weight loss. And you must contend with a food marketing environment that strongly promotes overeating. If you then regain the weight that you managed to lose, you are not alone. Most dieters gain back at least some of the lost weight.

The result has been a relentless search for an easier way to eat less, whether through diets, drugs, or surgery. For dieters the options appear infinite. For starters, we searched for "weight loss books" on Amazon.com, and up popped 16,000 titles. The intense interest in dieting books is nothing new. More than a century ago Sylvester Graham, John Harvey Kellogg, and Horace Fletcher had their cult followers, as do many of today's diet gurus. As the historian of diets Susan Yager explained in a cleverly oxymoronic subtitle, Americans have a "voracious appetite for losing weight."[11]

The first diet book based on calorie counting that we have been able to find appeared in 1918, less than twenty years after Wilbur Atwater brought calories to public attention. Drawing on Atwater's work, a physician, Lulu Hunt Peters, wrote *Diet and Health with Key to the Calories*, whose title pays homage to Mary Baker Eddy's *Science and Health with Key to the Scriptures*. What calorie counting might have to do with Baker Eddy's Christian Science philosophy is unclear. Peters dedicated her book to Herbert Hoover, who was then head of the U.S. Food Administration and responsible for its slogan, "Food will win the war." A phenomenal best seller at the time, Peters's book had gone through seventeen editions by 1922.[12]

It is easy to understand its popularity. Peters is fun to read, and the book is illustrated with charming stick-figure drawings from her 12-year-old nephew. Even today her advice sounds remarkably familiar: "You may eat just what you like—candy, pie, cake, fat meat, butter cream—but—*count your calories.* You can't have many nor large helpings, you see; but isn't it comforting to know that you can eat these things? Maybe some meal you would rather have a 350-calorie piece of luscious pie, with a delicious 150-calorie tablespoonful of whipped cream on it, than all the succulent vegetables Luther Burbank could grow in California. . . . Now that you know you can have the things you like, proceed to make your menus containing very little of them."[13]

In 1930, in an effort to educate the public about the still rather new concept of calories, USDA home economists published posters such as the one shown in figure 15. This illustrates 100-calorie portions of a variety of commonly consumed foods. Because portion sizes have increased so dramatically over the years, a poster like this today would need to display examples of 100-calorie fractions of typical servings: two Oreo cookies, one-third of a small hamburger, one-fifth of a bagel.

These days the most popular diet books have similar "eat less" goals but hardly ever discuss calories. Instead, they complicate the message by advising the restriction of one or another food group or component. Early in 2011, Amazon.com's best-selling weight loss book was *The 4-Hour Body: An Uncommon Guide to Rapid Fat-Loss, Incredible Sex, and Becoming Super-human*, by Timothy Ferriss (Crown Archetype, 2010). Never mind the title, the photographs of body builders, or the promises to women of fifteen-minute orgasms. One aspect of its dietary advice is right on target: "Don't drink your calories."

But even the most casual glance at perennial best-selling diet books can confuse any dieter. The books promote principles that thoroughly contradict one another: low fat vs. low carbohydrate, meat vs. vegetables, counting calories vs. ignoring them. Take your pick. If these diets help people reduce calorie intake below expenditure, any of them should work—for as long as dieters stick to them.

Sticking to the diet is the crucial issue. Most weight-loss studies find that 80 to 95 percent of dieters who manage to lose weight also manage to gain most of it back within a year or two. In 2010, researchers reported the weight maintenance results of the 1999–2006 National Health and Nutrition Examination Survey (NHANES). About 17 percent of dieters were able

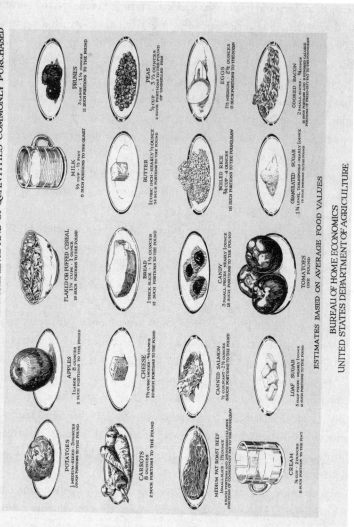

FIGURE 15. USDA poster illustrating 100-calorie portions, 1930. Foods typically consumed by Americans during the Depression are displayed on what must be 5-inch plates. USDA home economists based the calorie counts on Wilbur Atwater's studies as expanded by subsequent investigators. (Source: National Archives, Washington, DC.)

to maintain a 10 percent weight loss for a year. This may sound optimistic but it means that the other 83 percent of dieters could not. A review of 29 studies of people enrolled in weight loss programs produced more complicated results. After five years the average weight loss among the people available for follow-up (many were not) was 3 percent of their initial body weights. Individuals who kept off more than that were more likely to have lost more than 40 pounds, to have been on very-low-calorie diets, to be exercising regularly, and to have received intensive counseling and support—key principles of successful dieting.[14]

Statistics notwithstanding, some dieters do lose weight and keep it off. Rena Wing and James Hill have enrolled at least 5,000 successful dieters—those who maintained at least a 30-pound weight loss for a year or more—in a National Weight Control Registry. Wing and Hill are using this cohort to identify the common factors that contribute to successful weight loss—at least in this particular self-selected group. And what might those be? People in their cohort reported eating a low-fat diet, monitoring their food intake and body weight, and being highly active.[15] In our view, this boils down to nothing more complicated than *eating less* and *moving more.*

How successful dieters manage to eat less, however, varies among individuals. Some restrict certain kinds of foods or limit food quantity. Others count calories. Whatever they do, they monitor their weight closely and eat less when they start to put on a few pounds. About half of the successful dieters report that they lost weight on their own, but others, especially women, said that it helped to be enrolled in commercial weight loss programs. Such programs typically provide highly structured eating patterns along with extensive counseling support.

But does restricting certain kinds of foods or food components make it easier to lose weight and keep it off? In the early stages of dieting, it most certainly does. Restricting carbohydrate intake causes rapid depletion of glycogen along with its bound water, an instantaneous weight loss that can amount to five pounds or so.[16] In later stages of dieting, however, the composition of the diet matters much less, as we explain next.

CHAPTER 19

Are All Calories Created Equal?

Whether the particular mix of protein, fat, and carbohydrate in a diet makes any difference to weight loss is not a new question. In 1964 a group from the Institute for Medical Research in Oakland, California, examined precisely this issue in case studies of five obese patients who resided in a hospital metabolic ward. The researchers fed each patient a liquid-formula diet containing the same number of calories per day—either 800, 850, or 1,200, depending on the patient, for ten weeks or more. Every three or four weeks the investigators changed the formula to vary its content of protein (from 14 to 36 percent of calories), fat (12 to 83 percent), and carbohydrate (3 to 64 percent). For example, a patient received 1,200 calories a day, from each of the three diets in turn. At the extremes, the diets provided 14 or 34 percent of the calories from protein, 13 or 83 percent from fat, and 3 or 60 percent from carbohydrate, as shown in table 20.

The title of the published report of the study summarized its results: "Calories Do Count." All of the obese patients lost weight at a constant rate, regardless of the composition of the diet. It did not matter whether the fat or carbohydrate was extremely high or low. The graph of their weight loss looked much like that of the fasting men shown in figure 12 (chapter 13). At first the patients lost weight quite rapidly, reflecting the loss of glycogen and its accompanying fluid. After that the rate of weight loss stayed relatively constant. Although this study involved only five subjects, it was conducted under rigidly controlled conditions of hospitalization. Even more important, the

TABLE 20   VARIATIONS IN THE COMPOSITION OF
ONE PATIENT'S 1,200-CALORIE WEIGHT-LOSS DIET,
PERCENT OF TOTAL CALORIE INTAKE

Days on diet	Protein	Fat	Carbohydrate
33	34	52	14
28	27	13	60
21	14	83	3

SOURCE: Kinsell et al., 1964:198 (see note 1).

study involved measurements—not estimates—of calories and body weights. We think its mid-twentieth-century conclusions remain unchallenged:

Weight changes appeared to bear no relationship to such changes in nutrients, so long as the caloric intake remained constant. None of the foregoing is intended to suggest that relatively high fat, high protein diets may not have certain desirable features in regimens designed to prevent weight gain or to produce actual weight loss. There is good reason to believe that the satiety value of such diets is superior to diets high in carbohydrate and low in fat, and hence, may be associated with better dietary adherence. Unfortunately, many obese individuals . . . tend to go on "carbohydrate binges," regardless of the theoretically greater satiety value of a high fat regimen.[1]

In the next chapter we will address whether one kind of diet or another really is any better at promoting satiety and adherence among people who are living in the real world and not under study in metabolic wards. In this chapter we deal with calories in general and those from carbohydrates in particular.

Our favorite recent example of "calories do count" is the widely publicized Twinkie diet experiment conducted in 2010 by a professor at Kansas State University. He lost 27 pounds over the course of 10 weeks, during which he reported eating nothing but a Hostess Twinkie every 3 hours and occasional snacks of Doritos chips, sugary cereals, and Oreo cookies. How could he lose weight on a junk food diet like this? He reduced his usual dietary intake by about 800 calories a day. As Dr. David Katz commented, "The most salient takeaway message from this N-of-1 [single subject] experiment is a message I routinely deliver already: calories count."[2]

Katz went on to say that the Twinkie experiment "pretty emphatically rebuts claims in such works as *Good Calories, Bad Calories* by Gary Taubes, which suggests that the role of calories in weight is subordinate to the source of calories." As Katz noted, the question of whether all calories are equal is a persistent one, and many popular diet regimes have been based on the idea that low-carbohydrate diets are particularly beneficial. In 2007, for example, the Atkins (low-carbohydrate, high-protein-and-fat) diet was so popular that supermarkets created special "low carb" sections. These were filled with supposedly low-carbohydrate pasta, bread, and snacks, but also high-calorie (but no-carbohydrate) items such as salad oils.

LOW-CARBOHYDRATE (AND, THEREFORE, HIGH-FAT) DIETS

Food carbohydrates come in two forms: complex (starches) and simple (sugars). Both are largely digested to—and absorbed as—glucose, the sugar in blood that provides fuel for the brain. Glucose is also metabolized for energy elsewhere in the body, and large excesses are stored as body fat. Low-carbohydrate diets have been around for decades, especially as popularized by Drs. Irwin Stillman and Robert Atkins.[3] Their plans were designed to mimic the stage of starvation in which carbohydrates are depleted and fat breaks down rapidly to supply energy. As we discussed in chapter 13, this situation causes excess fatty acids to be converted into ketones. These circulate in blood and can be used by the brain as fuel when glucose is insufficient. When ketones reach high enough levels in blood, they can vaporize and be smelled in exhaled breath.

Since the early 2000s, numerous clinical trials have evaluated the effectiveness of low-carbohydrate diets for weight loss. As with all weight-loss trials, these report that participants lose weight within the first six months but then gain some of it back. Some—but not all—studies of low-carbohydrate diets have observed improvements in metabolic markers for chronic disease such as blood pressure, blood glucose levels, and blood lipid profiles. Typically, these studies lasted for only short periods and experienced high dropout rates.[4]

More important for this discussion, the studies rarely collected information about calorie intake. When they did get this information, it was through self-reports. Weight loss is a "hard" end point, meaning that it can be measured accurately. Self-reported calorie information, on the other hand, is unreliable and "soft." Because of such sources of error, it is not possible to know whether the weight loss and improved metabolic markers found in these studies were due to the low carbohydrate composition of the diet or to a reduced calorie intake.

Very-low-carbohydrate, high-fat diets may be satiating, but they are not especially healthy (they are low in fiber and some vitamins, for example), and ketosis is not pleasant to endure. Bad breath can be a typical symptom, as can other minor problems such as headaches. These go away when carbohydrate is reintroduced into the diet.[5]

THE GLYCEMIC INDEX (GI)

We trace more scientific interest in low-carbohydrate diets to studies in the 1980s by David Jenkins at the University of Toronto. Jenkins proposed a new term, the *glycemic index* (GI), as a way to differentiate sources of food carbohydrates and their effects on blood glucose.[6] High-GI foods—those with sugars and other rapidly digested and absorbed starches such as those in refined white flour—cause a rapid rise in blood glucose levels. Low-GI foods—those higher in protein, fat, and less rapidly digestible carbohydrates (whole grain and other fiber-containing foods, for example)—cause a slower and shallower rise in blood glucose that persists for a longer time. Eating low-GI foods could help people who have diabetes—a disease of insulin insufficiency (type 1) or cellular resistance to insulin (type 2)—to avoid large spikes in blood glucose levels after meals.

Spikes in blood glucose cause a rapid rise in secretion of insulin by the pancreas. Insulin, among other actions, increases the uptake of glucose by the brain, muscle, and adipose tissue, stimulates fatty acid storage, and inhibits fat mobilization from adipose tissue. Eating high-GI foods causes insulin levels to rise rapidly but also to fall rapidly once glucose is taken up by the tissues. This can make people feel hungrier and stimulate overeating. In contrast, after eating a low-GI meal, the hormonal responses are not as extreme. On this basis, David Ludwig and his colleagues propose that habitual eating of high-GI foods increases the risk of obesity and its consequences.[7]

LOW-CARBOHYDRATE ADVOCACY

Drawing on such ideas, the journalist Gary Taubes goes so far as to say that carbohydrates alone are responsible for obesity and that it is impossible to gain weight on low-carbohydrate diets irrespective of how many calories they contain. He comes to this conclusion on the basis of the way carbohydrates induce the pancreas to secrete insulin. When insulin levels are high, fat deposits do not break down to supply energy, and the effects of food are not as satiating. Taubes concludes that obesity is a disorder of excessively high insulin and excess fat accumulation. Excess intake of calories, he says, does not cause children to grow fatter any more than it causes them to grow taller. Obesity, he says, "is caused by the quality of the calories rather than the quantity, and specifically by the effect of refined and easily digestible carbohydrates on the hormonal regulation of fat storage and metabolism."[8]

As part of the evidence for this view, Taubes cites studies concluding that obese people do not eat more calories than those who are lean. But such studies, as we discussed in chapter 10, typically rely on self-reports of dietary intakes. More careful studies, particularly those done with doubly labeled water, make it clear that heavier people eat more calories than their lean counterparts but tend to underreport their calorie intake to a greater extent. The Institute of Medicine reviewed studies using the newer techniques and concluded that people with higher body weights do indeed eat more calories.[9]

Critical reviewers of Taubes's work praise its useful information, engaging writing, and insistence that something urgently needs to be done to get people to cut down on sugary sodas and eat fewer desserts. On the other hand, they criticize Taubes's reductionist view that obesity—a complex problem resulting from the interaction of genetics and behavior and affected by an exceptionally large number of hormonal and other regulatory factors—is largely due to a single cause: the effects of carbohydrate on insulin.[10]

THE ROLE OF FRUCTOSE

Taubes draws on another line of evidence for his emphasis on carbohydrates having to do with fructose, the sugar naturally found in fruit. Fructose is sweeter than glucose. Biochemically, fructose constitutes about 50 percent of sucrose (table sugar) and 55 percent of high fructose corn syrup (HFCS), sweeteners consumed in the United States in increasingly large amounts. In 1980, at the dawn of the obesity epidemic, the U.S. food supply provided 120 pounds of added caloric sweeteners per capita per year—84 pounds from sucrose, 35 pounds from HFCS, and the rest from honey and maple syrup. By 2008 the total had increased to 136 pounds per year, but the mix had changed.

The amount of sucrose in the food supply decreased by 18 pounds, but this decline was more than offset by a 34-pound increase in HFCS, which has the same number of calories as sucrose. Fructose, we must emphasize, comprises about half of both sweeteners (glucose is the other half).[11]

Nobody is or should be worried about the fructose in fruit, because fruits do not have all that much, and whatever fructose they do have is accompanied by fiber, vitamins, minerals, antioxidants, and other good things. Added fructose is another matter. Much fructose is consumed in sweetened beverages—fruit juices, fruit drinks, and sodas. These now account for more than 20 percent of daily calories among Americans, which is why advice to "stop drinking your calories" makes good sense. Some estimates suggest that fructose alone now provides about 10 percent of the calories consumed in the United States and as much as 12 percent of the calories consumed by adolescents. Among adolescents, 20 percent are thought to consume 25 percent or more of their total calories as fructose.[12] And the fructose in sodas and many other sweetened drinks is accompanied by an equal amount of highly available and rapidly absorbable glucose.

Beyond quantity, what most concerns medical experts about fructose is the way it is metabolized.[13] Dietary glucose raises blood glucose levels and causes the release of insulin, which gets the sugar into body cells and the brain and eventually turns off hunger signals. Fructose does not. Dietary fructose is transported directly to the liver, where some of it can be converted to glucose. But when large amounts are consumed, fructose is mostly metabolized to fat (triglycerides). Excessive fructose raises blood triglyceride levels, a characteristic feature of the metabolic syndrome we discussed in chapter 16 and a risk factor for cardiovascular disease. Fructose is also linked to non-alcoholic fatty liver disease (NAFLD), a condition rising in prevalence in parallel with rising rates of obesity. The metabolism of excess fructose is quite similar to the metabolism of alcohol, and increasing evidence suggests that the fatty livers that occur in response to an excess of either alcohol or fructose have a common metabolic origin.[14]

Researchers have increasingly linked the consumption of fructose-laden sugary drinks to obesity, especially among children. Liquid calories—those from alcoholic beverages and sweetened drinks—do not seem to have the same effect on satiety signals as those from food. In addition to weight gain and obesity, studies find sweetened beverages to be closely associated with the metabolic syndrome and type 2 diabetes.[15]

What should you make of all this? Carbohydrate calories are no different from any other type, although the body appears to have more difficulty regulating the intake of liquid sugars in general and metabolizing large amounts of fructose sugar in particular. Excessive fructose is metabolized differently than glucose, and the difference may induce harm. We have no doubt that cutting down on sugars and rapidly absorbable starches is an effective way for many people to reduce their calorie intake, resolve issues related to insulin spikes, and maybe even lose weight. And we thoroughly agree that people would be much better off eating whole grain starches, consuming sweets in smaller amounts, and reserving sugary drinks for special occasions. If nothing else, these choices would help reduce calorie intake.

Under tightly controlled hospital conditions, the source of calories makes no difference in weight loss. But what happens when people are not locked up in hospital metabolic wards? Do they lose weight better on low-carbohydrate diets, and do such diets help them keep the weight off? In the next chapter we take a look at studies comparing the effects of various kinds of weight-loss diets on people who live in the real world.

CHAPTER 20

Do Some Kinds of Diets
Work Better than Others?

One problem in studying the effects of dietary composition is that it is not possible to vary the proportion of one component without changing the others. At the extremes of weight-loss diets, the Atkins and South Beach diets are low carbohydrate but high fat, while the Ornish diet is low fat, high carbohydrate.[1] To compare the effects of such diets outside metabolic wards, researchers must deal with study subjects whose dietary and other behaviors are not easily controlled.

Investigators do everything they can to encourage compliance with study protocols. But they confront a major challenge: telling free-living people what you want them to eat does not necessarily mean that they will follow your instructions or tell you the truth about what they are eating. And you have no easy way of getting around this problem. Because dietary intake methods all depend on accurately disclosing what subjects consume—something impossible for most people to do—the lack of an easy way to measure true calorie consumption in weight control studies must be considered "the fundamental flaw of obesity research."[2]

But that's not the only problem. When conducting clinical trials that compare one diet to another, researchers also face challenges in enrolling enough study subjects to satisfy statistical requirements, getting study subjects to stick to the prescribed diets, and retaining participants in the study throughout its length. Furthermore, clinical trials of diet and weight loss are expensive to conduct, and few are able to last long enough to observe whether initial weight losses were regained. These considerations make it especially difficult for investigators to evaluate the results of dietary studies objectively and for others to interpret the significance of the findings. Keep these caveats in mind as we take a look at some of the studies attempting to find out whether varying the proportions of protein, fat, and carbohydrate makes any difference to weight loss in real life.

LOW-FAT (AND, THEREFORE, HIGH-CARBOHYDRATE) DIETS

Atwater Values indicate that fat has more than twice the energy value of either protein or carbohydrate. It makes sense to think that cutting down on fat would help with weight maintenance or loss. In the United States the various editions of the Dietary Guidelines have long promoted lower-fat diets: "Avoid too much fat" (1980, 1985), "Choose a diet low in fat" (1990, 1995), "Keep total fat intake between 20 to 35 percent of calories" (2005), and "Reduce intake of solid fats" (2010). The more recent editions have focused on limiting saturated fat and cholesterol intake rather than total fat per se in recognition of the potential role of these components in heart disease risk. But the newer guidelines also recognize that from the standpoint of body weight, calories from fat are no different from calories from any other source.

This is a shift from earlier recommendations that reshaped the marketplace. In the early 1990s, advice to reduce fat intake was all that food companies needed to hear to start making low-fat versions of many common foods—low-fat cheese, mayonnaise, and peanut butter, for example—along with oxymoronic products such as fat-free "dairy" creamer and fat-free (but equally caloric) cookies. Such products are not necessarily healthier than the products they replace and rarely taste as good.

But the relationship of dietary fat to obesity is still of much interest. For one thing, it takes hardly any energy to store excess fatty acids as body fat, whereas it takes a bit more energy to make fatty acids from excess dietary carbohydrate. For another, proponents of low-fat diets cite experimental observations demonstrating a connection between fat intake and overweight:

+ Laboratory animals fed high-fat diets generally become obese.
+ Populations consuming low-fat diets maintain lower body weights.
+ Some clinical studies show that reducing dietary fat can result in modest weight loss.[3]

Some experts, however, view such evidence as not at all specific to fat, as it could just as easily relate to high-calorie diets from any source. Low-fat diets are necessarily high in carbohydrate—the calories have to come from something—and few studies control for total calories consumed. Overall, studies of dietary patterns typically find no association between either the amount or the type of fat in the diet and subsequent weight gain over periods of several years.[4]

When investigators compare the effects of weight-loss diets varying in fat content, they find little difference. One study, for example, looked at overweight or obese subjects who had reduced their body weights by about 25 pounds by consuming a diet of 800 calories a day—a reduction that ought to induce weight loss in anyone. The participants were divided into groups and instructed to consume specified diets containing 20 to 45 percent of calories from fat. Because all participants regained weight at about the same rate during the study period, the investigators concluded that the percentage of dietary fat made no difference.[5]

Another study, this one of nearly 50,000 women, compared the effects of low-fat to usual diets over a six-year period. The women assigned to the low-fat diet were treated more attentively and perhaps for this reason lost more weight during the first year. They also had lower levels of body fat. Those who best adhered to the low-fat diet kept the weight off the longest. But by the end of the study period, the difference between the two groups was too small to be statistically significant. The one long-term benefit seen in the women on the low-fat diet was a small decrease in body fat.[6] Was this benefit due to the low-fat intake or to the reduction in calories? Our guess is fewer calories.

HIGH-PROTEIN (AND USUALLY HIGH-FAT) DIETS

Diets are limited in the amount of protein they contain because most foods do not have much. Even a lean beef steak is only 25 percent protein by weight (the rest is water and fat), and this works out to less than 40 percent of its calories. Typical mixed diets provide only 10 to 15 percent of calories from protein. In Wilbur Atwater's energy scheme, the value of protein, 4 calories per gram, is the same as that for carbohydrate. As we discussed in chapter 7, eating protein produces greater heat losses in metabolism (20 to 30 percent of the initial calories) than eating sugars (5 to 10 percent) or fat (0 to 5 percent). Thermic effects suggest that high-protein diets might be good choices for weight loss since protein calories are used less efficiently.

In practice, however, the difference in thermic effects turns out to be small. A study in which up to 18 percent of carbohydrate was replaced with protein found energy expenditure to increase by only about 3 percent. After reviewing published studies of the thermic effects of diets varying in protein, investigators from Tufts University developed equations to predict the number of calories lost as heat in response to diets of varying composition. These equations estimate that the difference in thermic effects of diets containing 15 percent and 30 percent protein would amount to just 23 calories a day.[7] If you reduce calorie intake by 500 to 1,000 calories a day, the difference in calories lost by eating a little more protein will be negligible. And protein-rich foods such as meat and beans tend to be relatively high in calories for their weight.

Are high-protein diets more satiating? A review of studies examining this question concluded unhelpfully that because the experiments produced such inconsistent results, more research would be needed to answer it.[8]

COMPARATIVE STUDIES

In 2001 a review of several of the most popular diets at that time, including the Atkins, Ornish, and Weight Watchers (point-counting) programs, found all of them to result in weight loss, provided that calories did not exceed 1,400 to 1,500 per day. Calorie balance, it concluded, was the major determinant of weight loss. All low-calorie diets help people lose weight, regardless of the proportions of protein, fat, and carbohydrate, and all reduce hunger and are satiating to a similar extent.[9]

Of the great many studies that have attempted to evaluate the comparative effects of dietary composition on weight loss, we think some of the longer-lasting trials with large numbers of subjects are especially worth examination. In 2007, Christopher Gardner and his Stanford colleagues reported the results of a one-year clinical trial to compare the weight-loss effects of the Atkins (high fat), Ornish (low fat), Zone (low carbohydrate), and LEARN (lifestyle behavior change) diets on about 300 overweight women. When the year was over, those on the Atkins diet had lost the most weight—an average of 10 pounds as compared to 6 pounds for those on other diets.[10]

Weight loss for the Atkins group was highest at six months, but participants soon began to regain weight. The investigators admitted that "longer follow-up would likely have resulted in progressively diminished group differences." They also noted that adherence "waned over time, especially for

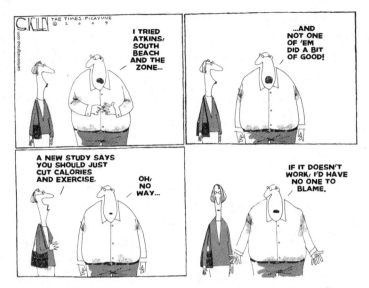

FIGURE 16. Diet confusion. From a dieter's standpoint, the inability to tell whether one or another diet will make any difference to weight loss is not particularly helpful. © Steve Kelley, used with permission of Steve Kelley and Creators Syndicate. All rights reserved.

the Atkins and Ornish diets," suggesting that many people find it difficult to eat extreme diets of one kind or another. Figure 16 illustrates one dieter's frustration with adherence to diets of any kind.

The Stanford study focused on diet composition, but the investigators collected as much information as they could about calorie intake through 24-hour recalls conducted by telephone. Participants in all four diet groups reported consuming 1,500 to 1,600 calories a day but with a possible range of plus or minus 400 to 500 calories—a rather large variation. Given the unreliability of such information, we cannot conclude that the Atkins diet was responsible for the transiently better weight loss or even that diets high in fat encourage people not to eat so much. To be meaningful, such studies must obtain accurate information about calorie intake, something inconvenient and expensive to do with large numbers of study subjects.

Other studies are difficult to compare and interpret, as they were done for different purposes using different protocols and study populations. In 2009, for example, investigators published the results of a study designed to determine whether differences in dietary composition might affect long-term compliance with weight-loss regimens. The study compared four diets:

- *low fat, average protein:* 20 percent fat, 15 percent protein, 65 percent carbohydrate
- *low fat, high protein:* 20 percent fat, 25 percent protein, 55 percent carbohydrate
- *high fat, average protein:* 40 percent fat, 15 percent protein, 45 percent carbohydrate
- *high fat, high protein:* 40 percent fat, 25 percent protein, 35 percent carbohydrate[11]

About 200 people were instructed to follow each of these dietary patterns for two years and to eat meals that reduced calorie intake by 750 a day. Nearly 80 percent of the initial participants completed the study. Those that did had an average weight loss of 9 pounds, and 15 percent lost at least 10 percent of their body weight. Most of the weight loss took place in the first six months. All groups reported similar levels of satiety, hunger, and diet satisfaction, and all showed improvements in fasting insulin levels and blood lipids.

The investigators estimated that the participants reduced their calorie intake by about 225 calories a day during the first six months, not 750. After the first year many of the participants regained some of the weight they had lost. On this basis, the researchers concluded that any reduced-calorie diet could result in "clinically meaningful" weight loss regardless of its protein, fat, and carbohydrate composition.

Proponents of low-carbohydrate diets would argue that this study did not really test the low-carbohydrate hypothesis—35 percent carbohydrate is not all that low. In 2010 a different group of investigators reported the results of a large clinical trial comparing the effectiveness of several diets in 773 obese volunteers in eight European countries. Their idea was to compare the effects of diets containing foods with a low or a high glycemic index (GI) in preventing weight gain after weight loss. The participants initially lost weight on diets of just 800 to 1,000 calories a day from a commercial weight-loss formula to which was added nearly a pound of vegetables. They lost an impressive average of 24 pounds.[12]

At that point they were assigned to one of five diets differing in the proportion of protein and carbohydrate and in foods with a high or a low GI and instructed to maintain the weight loss. During the next six months the participants gained back some of the weight they had lost. The largest regain, four pounds, was observed in the group consuming the high-GI, low-protein diet. The weights of those on the low-GI diet stayed about the same. This was a short-term study that ended six months after the initial weight loss, so it is difficult to say what would have happened had it continued. A more serious problem was that 29 percent of the participants dropped out before the end of the study, although the lowest dropout rate occurred among those on the low-GI, high-protein diet, suggesting some value to this approach.

Also in 2010, three medical centers in the United States collaborated on a comparison of low-carbohydrate and low-fat diets. The investigators asked half of 300 obese volunteers with an average BMI of 36 to consume a relatively low-fat diet and to limit calorie intake to 1,200 to 1,500 a day for women and 1,500 to 1,800 for men. *Relatively low-fat* in this case means 30 percent of calories, an amount that is not especially low. The investigators assigned the other half of the participants to an Atkins-type diet that limited carbohydrate but allowed unrestricted consumption of fat and protein. The groups received extensive counseling to encourage adherence to the diets.[13]

Both groups had lost about 11 percent of their initial weight after one year. By two years, the total loss was still 7 percent. The investigators concluded that the two diets produced the same energy deficit in both groups and that successful weight loss could be achieved with either diet when it was coupled with behavioral treatment. We wish they had reported calorie measurements, but they did not.

Complicating the interpretation of this study is that its dropout rate was exceptionally high. Despite intensive counseling, 32 percent of participants in the "low"-fat regimen and 46 percent of those on the low-carbohydrate Atkins-type diet failed to complete the trial. If nothing else, this study demonstrated how difficult it is for many people to stick to diets in general and to low-carbohydrate diets in particular. Those who did stay on the low-carbohydrate diet improved their blood cholesterol profiles, thereby reducing some risk factors for coronary heart disease.

But some critics of low-carbohydrate diets have raised questions about their long-term effects on health. The data from a large prospective study of men and women who had been followed for more than twenty years suggest that if a low-carbohydrate diet includes large amounts of animal protein (meat), it is associated with a slight *increase* in mortality. But if the low-carbohydrate diet includes large amounts of vegetables, mortality is reduced. In this study, reported carbohydrate levels ranged from about 30 to 55 percent of calories. The investigators did not say whether reported calorie intakes or body weights changed during the course of the study, so the role of calories in these results is unknown.[14]

Every five years a committee of the Departments of Health and Human Services (HHS) and Agriculture (USDA) produces the Dietary Guidelines advisory report, which represents mainstream, science-based consensus on dietary advice. Although, as Marion Nestle discussed in her book *Food Politics*, such committees are not always free of political influence, this particular group went to unusual efforts to evaluate the science as objectively as possible, and we consider its views to be reasonably authoritative.

In its massive review of studies of diet and weight loss, the 2010 Dietary Guidelines Advisory Committee concluded, "No optimal macronutrient [protein, fat, carbohydrate] proportion was identified for enhancing weight loss or weight maintenance. However, decreasing caloric intake led to increased weight loss and improved weight maintenance. . . . Diets that are less than 45 percent carbohydrate or more than 35 percent protein are difficult to adhere to, are not more effective than other calorie-controlled diets for weight loss and weight maintenance, and may pose health risk, and are therefore not recommended for weight loss or maintenance."[15]

Overall, the comparative studies to date demonstrate that study participants find it easier to gain weight than to lose it and easier to lose weight than to keep it off. Jeffrey Friedman believes that the effects of regulatory signals such as leptin help to explain these difficulties.[16] As we explained in chapter 12, deliberate weight loss opposes a physiological system designed to promote eating and to discourage semistarvation or even milder dieting. A food environment that encourages overeating can easily get around the system's weak stop signals. Some people can handle the temptations of an "eat more" food environment and remain relatively thin, but many others cannot and find it all too easy to consume more calories than they need.

The source of the calories may make a small difference in weight maintenance or loss, but it appears to be much less important than the ability to resist pressures to overeat calories in general. Our personal preference is for diets that provide plenty of fruits, vegetables, fish or lean meats, and whole grains and that avoid sugary drinks and minimize high-calorie snacks. This kind of diet is useful for overall health reasons and should also help with weight maintenance.

We have repeatedly referred to environmental reasons for regaining weight after dieting. As Dr. David Kessler explains in *The End of Overeating*, the pleasure you get from consuming high-calorie foods full of salt, sugar, and fat overrides biological regulatory signals by rewiring your brain to cause you to want to eat more of those foods. The food industry, he suggests, has taken advantage of this vulnerability by marketing foods that induce you to consume more calories than you need.[17] How this happens comes next.

PART SIX

The Politics of Calories

A Closer Look

In previous sections we have explained how politics—as well as science—affects views of the role of calories in the diets of individuals and groups. Of course calories are affected by politics. As with everything else having to do with food and nutrition, many different groups have a stake in how calories are marketed, perceived, labeled, and promoted. The chapters in this last section deal with specific aspects of the social and political environment of calories, beginning with the ways in which this environment has changed. We view the results of these changes, many of which occurred as inadvertent responses to greater food production and competition in the food industry, as strongly promoting the overconsumption of calories. In some ways, the calorie environment could not have been more brilliantly constructed to overcome physiological controls of overeating. In today's "eat more" environment, attempts to balance calorie intake against expenditure face powerful opposing forces. These forces are particularly difficult to overcome because calories in food are so misperceived. Most people cannot estimate their calorie intake or expenditure with anywhere near the accuracy needed to consciously control calorie balance effectively.

The opposing forces seem even more powerful in the light of evidence that education about the food environment is rarely enough to change behavior. Even people who are taught that larger food portions encourage overeating will overeat when presented with large plates of food. But surely information about calories on food labels ought to help individuals make better choices? In the chapters in this section we discuss the FDA's calorie labeling regulations and the reasons why the calories in alcoholic beverages rarely appear on their labels. In both instances, regulatory agencies must contend with industries that greatly prefer not to label calories and agree to do so only when forced or, occasionally, when doing so seems to serve their interests.

In recent years the FDA has proposed to improve package labeling, the USDA has enacted new labeling initiatives for meat and poultry, and Congress has passed a law requiring chain restaurants to post calories on menu boards. Early research on the value of such initiatives has yielded mixed results. The studies show that calorie information improves knowledge to some extent but, as is often the case with educational initiatives, has little immediate effect on behavior. Whether these initiatives will have beneficial effects in the long term is still unknown. Education ought to help people overcome basic biological drives to eat in the context of an "eat more" food environment, but it is likely to be most effective when supported by environmental changes that promote healthier patterns of diet and physical activity.

CHAPTER 21

Today's "Eat More" Environment
The Role of the Food Industry

Weight gain, as we keep saying, is caused by eating more, moving less, or doing both. Rates of overweight and obesity began to rise sharply in the United States in the early 1980s. Did Americans start becoming less active at that time? Did they begin to eat more? Or, as is widely believed, did both things happen simultaneously? Let's take a look.

TREND: CALORIES EXPENDED IN PHYSICAL ACTIVITY

Practically anyone you ask will tell you that people in general and kids in particular are less active now than they were in recent decades. Kids hardly ever take physical education classes, walk or ride bicycles to school, or play spontaneous sports. If enrolled in organized sports, they spend more time hanging around than running around. You cannot tear them away from computers, video games, or other sedentary online entertainment. On this basis, some researchers insist that declining levels of physical activity—not eating more calories—must be the chief cause of today's obesity crisis.[1]

We wish we had compelling reasons to believe this idea to be correct, but we do not. If anything, research shows the opposite. Doubly labeled water studies indicate a slight *increase* in physical activity since the early 1980s. Even research based on self-reports, which tend to exaggerate the most healthful practices, finds practically no change in calorie expenditures since 1980. The CDC, for example, conducts periodic surveys of physical activity levels

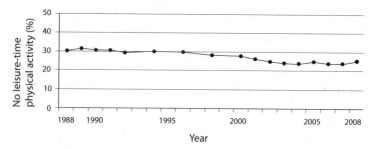

FIGURE 17. Rates of self-reported leisure-time inactivity, 1988–2008. If inactivity is declining slightly, activity levels must be increasing slightly. Source: CDC, 2010 (see note 2).

based on self-reports. These show a slight increase in reported activity levels from 1990 to 1998. The CDC also asks questions about leisure-time sedentary behavior. The responses indicate a slight decline in inactivity from 1988 to 2008, as shown in figure 17.[2]

Additional CDC surveys record small increases in physical activity among men and women from 2001 to 2005. But other investigators report slight decreases in activity and slight increases in inactivity among ninth- and tenth-grade boys and among both black and white girls between the ages of nine and nineteen. The studies finding such results used different methods, age groups, and time periods and are not easily compared. To try to make sense of the conflicting data, Australian investigators reviewed every study they could find on levels of physical activity but observed that almost none had collected baseline data on childhood activity from the earlier years. Without a baseline, they could not identify a trend.

They noted, however, that today's declining rates of active transport (walking, cycling), school physical education, and organized sports constitute what they call an "activity toxic" environment for kids. Kids want to be active but are constrained by school policies and curricula, parental concerns about safety and convenience, and the almost universal lack of sidewalks, bike paths, and safe places to play.[3]

Years ago kids were watching television and reading comic books. Are they really less active now? Without better data we cannot agree that declining physical activity is the more important cause of rising rates of overweight, especially because most data are self-reported. We did find one longitudinal

TABLE 21   TRENDS IN SELF-REPORTED CALORIE
INTAKE, 1971–2008, PER CAPITA PER DAY

Year	Men	Women
1971–1974	2,450	1,540
1976–1980	2,440	1,520
1988–1994	2,670	1,800
1999–2000	2,620	1,880
2001–2002	2,620	1,845
2003–2004	2,610	1,850
2005–2006	2,640	1,785
2007–2008	2,510	1,770

SOURCES: 1971–2000 figures are from National Health and Nutrition Examination Surveys of people ages 20–74 (CDC, 2004; see note 5); 2001–2008 figures come from *What We Eat in America* surveys, ages 20–74+ (USDA, 2010;
see note 6).
NOTE: Calories rounded off to the nearest 5.

study that measured baseline calorie intake and expenditure with doubly
labeled water. Baseline total energy intake and resting energy expenditure
predicted subsequent obesity, but energy expenditure from physical activity
did not.[4] Overall, the available evidence points to calorie intake as a more
important cause of obesity than calorie output.

TREND: CALORIE INTAKE

Studies of calorie intake are much less ambiguous. For them, we have baseline data. Compared to studies dating back to the early 1970s, recent studies
show a clear increase in calorie intake, as shown in table 21.[5]

These figures require some interpretation. They were obtained from self-
reports of one-day diet recalls, cover different age groups, may not represent average daily intake, and undoubtedly underreport calories. Taking the
results at face value, men in recent years reported eating about 200 more
calories per day than men in 1971–74. For women, the increase for the same
time period is more than 300 calories a day. Since 2000, reported calorie
intake has declined somewhat, possibly as a result of extending the age range
of participants (older people eat less). But whatever the exact number, calorie
intakes seem to have increased.[6] Why? To answer this question, let's look at
concurrent changes in the food environment.

CALORIES IN THE FOOD ENVIRONMENT

Since the early 1980s the U.S. food environment has changed in ways that encourage eating in more places at more times of day in larger portions.[7] We attribute these changes to food industry responses to a sharp increase in the number of calories available in the food supply. For more than seventy years, from the early 1900s to the early 1980s, the U.S. food supply provided an average of about 3,200 calories per person per day, with a variation of plus or minus 200 calories. But by 2000 the available calories had increased to 3,900 per person per day, in parallel with rising rates of obesity. We illustrate these trends in figure 18.

Although calories in the food supply have increased by 700 per person per day since 1980 or so, the constituent proportions of protein (11 percent of calories), fat (41 percent), and carbohydrate (48 percent) show no evident change during that period. The mix of sources within those categories also did not change, except for the replacement of some fats from meat and dairy products with those from liquid oils. Calories from proteins, fats, and carbohydrates increased in direct proportion to total calories.[8]

Nevertheless, the kinds of foods that deliver many of the calories to American diets are a matter of considerable concern. The National Health and Nutrition Examination Survey (NHANES) collects data on dietary intake that can be used to identify the foods that are leading sources of calories in American diets. Table 22 summarizes data from the 2005–2006 NHANES. The leading contributors are desserts (grain-based and dairy), sodas, pizza, chips, and burgers. Chicken appears as the number three source, no doubt because the category includes fried chicken and McNuggets. These are largely foods of low nutrient density and high calorie density—junk foods. Worse, the top *three* food sources of calories for children ages 2 to 18 are grain-based desserts (138 calories per day), pizza (136 calories), and sodas and energy and sports drinks (118 calories). Together these three food sources contribute one-fourth of a child's daily calorie intake. NHANES figures are national averages; some children obtain even more of their calories from such foods.[9]

Sugary drinks are of special concern. A later analysis of NHANES data from 2005 to 2008 reports that boys ages 12 to 19 consume nearly 300 calories a day from sugary drinks alone, and that 5 percent of the U.S. population consumes nearly 570 calories a day from such drinks. These contain sugars but no or few nutrients and are as low in nutrient density as you can get.[10]

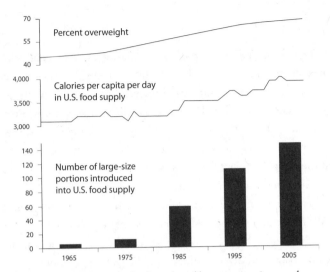

FIGURE 18. Calories in the food supply and large portions increased in tandem with rates of obesity from 1960 to 2005: trends in overweight (top panel), calories in the food supply per capita per day (middle panel), and introduction of larger food portions (bottom panel). Figure courtesy of Dr. Lisa Young.

TABLE 22   TOP 15 SOURCES OF CALORIES IN U.S. DIETS, PEOPLE AGES 2 AND OLDER

Rank	Calorie source	Calories per day from that source
1	Grain-based desserts (cakes, cookies, pies, donuts)	138
2	Yeast breads	129
3	Chicken and chicken mixed dishes	121
4	Sodas, energy and sports drinks, sweetened waters	114
5	Pizza	98
6	Alcoholic beverages	82
7	Pasta and pasta dishes	81
8	Tortillas, burritos, tacos, nachos	80
9	Beef and beef mixed dishes	64
10	Dairy desserts (ice cream, sherbet, pudding)	62
11	Chips: potato, corn, other	56
12	Burgers	53
13	Reduced-fat milk	51
14	Cheese	49
15	Ready-to-eat cereals	49

SOURCE: USDA, HHS, 2010 (see note 9).

The Causes

Why more calories became available is a matter of some conjecture. One frequently cited cause is the influx of women into the workforce, creating demands for convenience. But before blaming women for causing obesity, consider the labor statistics. These suggest that while women in the workforce—and longer working hours—may be contributing factors, the timing isn't quite right. By the early 1980s, half of working-age women had already entered the workforce, and from 1981 to 2007 the percentage only increased from 52 to 60 percent.[11] In any case, women can hardly be blamed for the food industry's creation of high-calorie, low-nutrient-density convenience foods. We think the evidence points more strongly to two other causes: agriculture policies and the advent of the "shareholder value" movement, which changed the way Wall Street evaluates publicly traded corporations.

Agricultural Policies. In 1973 and 1977, Congress passed laws that reversed long-standing farm policies aimed at protecting prices by controlling production. These policies paid farmers to set aside acres, but that changed when Earl Butz, a former dean of agriculture at Purdue, became USDA secretary and reportedly urged them to plant "fencerow to fencerow." Whether Butz really said this or not—no source has ever been found for the statement—the new policies encouraged farmers to plant as much as they possibly could. Food production increased, and so did calories in the food supply. The addition of 700 calories a day per capita made the food industry even more competitive. Food companies now had to find new ways to sell products in an environment that offered a vast excess of calories over the needs of the population. Even if, as the USDA maintains, Americans waste a third of available calories, the food supply is still highly overabundant.[12]

The "Shareholder Value" Movement. The onset of a movement to force corporations to produce more immediate and higher returns on investment especially increased competitive pressures on food companies. The movement's start is attributed to a speech given by Jack Welch, then head of General Electric, in 1981. Corporations, Welch said, owed more to their shareholders. His company would now focus on producing faster growth and higher profit margins and returns to investors. The movement caught on quickly, and Wall Street soon began to press companies to report not only profit but also increased *growth* on a quarterly basis. Food companies were having enough trouble producing profits in an overabundant food economy. Now they had to demonstrate profit growth every ninety days.[13]

The Consequences

Competitive pressures forced food companies to consolidate, become larger, and seek new markets and ways to expand sales in existing markets. The collateral result was a changed society. Today, in contrast to the early 1980s, it is socially acceptable to eat in more places, more frequently, and in larger amounts, and for children to regularly consume fast foods, snacks, and sodas—changes that singly and together promote higher calorie intakes. Here we highlight just a few of the ways in which the altered food environment promotes overeating.[14]

Foods away from Home. An abundance of food creates a cheap food supply, making it less expensive for people to eat foods prepared outside the home. Beginning in the late 1970s, spending on away-from-home foods rose from about one-third of total food expenditures to about one-half. The proportion of calories obtained from away-from-home foods rose from less than 20 to more than 30 percent, with much of the increase coming from fast food. Among children, the percentage of daily energy eaten away from home increased from 23 to 34 percent. According to an analysis of national food consumption surveys, children get more of their daily calories from fast-food outlets than they do from schools, and fast food is the largest contributor to the calories they consume outside the home. USDA economists say that the average meal eaten away from home by adults adds 134 calories to daily intakes, and one meal a week eaten at a restaurant can account for a two-pound annual weight gain.[15]

New Products. The low cost of basic food commodities has encouraged food companies to make new forms of tasty packaged food products. Manufacturers introduce nearly 20,000 new products into the food supply each year, nearly half of them candies, gums, snacks, and sodas. The habitual consumption of such foods is associated with long-term increases in calorie intake and body weight, and 40 percent of the calories in the diets of children and adolescents are reported to derive from high-calorie sweets and snack foods.[16]

Larger Portions. Once food became relatively cheap, restaurants, fast-food chains, and major food companies could offer foods and beverages in larger sizes to attract customers. Larger portions have more calories. They also encourage people to eat more and to underestimate the number of calories in their food by larger percentages. The increase in portion sizes is sufficient to explain rising levels of obesity (see figure 18).[17]

Ubiquity. We like to ask the question "When did it become acceptable to eat in bookstores?" Today snack foods are sold in 96 percent of pharmacies, 94 percent of gasoline stations, 22 percent of furniture stores, and 16 percent of apparel stores. Research shows that if food is at hand, people will eat it.[18]

Frequency. Nibbling may seem like a good idea, but the more times a day people eat junk foods, the more calories they are likely to consume. It now seems normal to snack and drink sodas throughout the day. Surveys find that children eat an average of three snacks per day, most of them high-calorie desserts, junk foods, and sweetened beverages of poor nutritional quality.[19]

Proximity. The mere location of fast-food restaurants near schools has been shown to promote fast-food consumption as well as overweight, even when corrected for community characteristics. Cornell professor Brian Wansink and his colleagues have demonstrated the calorie-promoting effects of having food close at hand. The closer the candy dish, the more candy consumed. The mere presence of vending machines encourages kids to buy high-calorie foods, which explains why health advocates would like to see vending machines removed from schools.[20]

Low Prices. Adam Drewnowski and his team at the University of Washington have shown that on a per-calorie basis, junk foods are cheaper than healthier foods. They estimate that following federal dietary advice to increase intake of fruits and vegetables would raise one's food costs by several hundred dollars a year. If fruits and vegetables appear more expensive than junk foods, it's because they are. The Consumer Price Index indicates an increase of about 40 percent in the relative cost of fruits and vegetables since the early 1980s, whereas the indexed price of desserts, snack foods, and sodas has declined by 20 to 30 percent. Lower prices encourage people to eat more. Higher prices discourage food purchases.[21] For example, as part of its contribution to obesity prevention, Coca-Cola now offers drinks in 7.5-ounce cans but prices them higher than 12-ounce sodas. As a retailing executive once explained to us, if customers want smaller portions, they ought to be willing to pay for them.

Marketing Health. The food industry spends billions of dollars a year to encourage people to buy its products, but foods marketed as "healthy" particularly encourage greater calorie intake. Professor Wansink's experiments show that people eat more calories from snack foods labeled low fat, no trans fat, or organic. Most people, he says, are "blissfully unaware" of how the food environment influences what they eat. People take in excessive calories "not because of hunger but because of family and friends, packages and plates, names and numbers, labels and lights, colors and candles, shapes and smells. . . . The list is almost as endless as it's invisible."[22]

Invisible to consumers, yes, but not to food marketers. The result of constant exposure to today's "eat more" food environment, as David Kessler explains in *The End of Overeating,* has been to drive people to desire high-calorie foods and to become "conditioned overeaters."[23] The power of this food environment to promote greater calorie intake is so great that even educated eaters have trouble dealing with it. If you as an educated eater have trouble managing "eat more" pressures it is because it is virtually impossible for individuals to judge the number of calories they are eating, as we discuss next.

CHAPTER 22

More Calorie Confusion

Portion Distortion, Health Halos, and Wishful Thinking

For many years Dr. Lisa Young, an expert on portion size and author of *The Portion Teller* (Crown, 2005), has taught an introductory nutrition class at New York University. As a favor to us, she agreed to devote some time on the first day of class to asking students about their basic understanding of food calories. Among her questions were these: How many calories are in an 8-ounce soda? How many calories are in a 64-ounce Double Gulp soda?

We did not expect beginning students to know the number of calories in an 8-ounce soft drink, and most did not. An 8-ounce soft drink contains about 100 calories. A drink 8 times larger should contain 8 times as many calories—800. Although this is not higher mathematics, only about a quarter of the class correctly multiplied the number they guessed for the size of the smaller drink by 8.

Instead, a large majority of students—nearly 70 percent—underestimated the calories in the larger drink. The underestimaters typically multiplied the calories in the 8-ounce drink by an average of 3, not 8. How could this be? We asked Dr. Young to try to find out from her students why their estimates were so far off. Their answer: 800 calories in a soda is *impossible*. They simply did not believe the math. Soda package labels, the students pointed out, never say "800 calories"; they say "100 calories per serving." Besides, drinking sodas doesn't make them feel full.

We should not have been surprised. In lectures, we often show a photograph of Dr. Young posed behind soft drink containers ranging from 8 to 64 ounces. When we tell audiences that a 64-ounce soda has 800 calories, we are met with gasps of disbelief—even from trained nutritionists. As we keep pointing out, calories are invisible and devoid of taste. You cannot tell how many are in a food just by looking at it or even tasting it. If you eat anything other than packaged foods with Nutrition Facts labels or anyplace other than fast-food restaurants that post calories on menu boards, you can only guess the number of calories in your foods. If you want to know how many calories you are eating, you have to weigh every ingredient in everything you eat and drink and look up the calories in food composition tables. Even so, these will only be estimates that depend on the accuracy of your weighing. Restaurant calories are particularly difficult because customers have no idea (and are not supposed to know) how the foods were prepared.

This is not because people are ignorant. Even professional nutritionists cannot estimate calories accurately. In the mid-1990s Marion Nestle and Lisa Young demonstrated this embarrassing fact when they were invited by *New York Times* reporter Marian Burros to lunch at a fine Italian restaurant in company with some other nutrition educators. Burros ordered two of everything on the menu. She asked the nutritionists to guess the calories in one set of meals and sent the matching meals off to a laboratory to be analyzed. Not one of the nutritionists came close to guessing that the small, lunch-size portion of risotto, for example, contained nearly 1,300 calories. These professional nutritionists underestimated the calories in those meals by about 30 percent.[1] Errors of that size are *typical*.

In another such experiment, Lisa Young asked dietitians attending an annual meeting of the American Dietetic Association to estimate the number of calories in samples of several fast-food meals. The dietitians accurately guessed the calories in a glass of whole milk but underestimated those in the mixed meals by the usual 30 percent or so. For example, when shown a typical chain-restaurant hamburger and onion rings, they guessed 865 calories on average, whereas the meal actually contained 1,550.[2]

Calorie estimations are especially inaccurate when the food portions are large and when the foods appear to be healthy, as researchers have repeatedly demonstrated.

THE PORTION SIZE EFFECT

Even students trained to know that portion size influences calorie estimations get fooled by large portions. Cornell professor Brian Wansink demonstrated this phenomenon in his famous Super Bowl experiment. He invited students to his home to watch a Super Bowl game. He put half of them in one room with 2-quart bowls of snacks and the other half in another room with 4-quart bowls. The students who were served snacks from the larger bowls consumed about 50 percent more calories than those served from the smaller bowls. Both groups underestimated the calories they had eaten, but those served the larger portions underestimated by a much larger proportion.[3]

These students should have known better. Even though they had heard lectures from Professor Wansink about the influence of large portions on the amount of food people consume, they ate more from the larger bowls anyway. And so does almost everyone else when confronted with large food portions.

THE "HEALTH HALO" EFFECT

People tend to underestimate the calories in foods that they perceive as healthy. This has led researchers to suggest that health claims cause a systematic bias in calorie perception.[4] Brian Wansink and his colleagues call this the health halo effect. We think of all such marketing methods as calorie distracters. Whatever you want to call the phenomenon, much evidence indicates that marketing a product as healthy makes people think it has fewer calories:

+ When fast-food restaurants position themselves as healthy, customers tend to underestimate the calories in main dishes and choose higher-calorie side dishes, drinks, or desserts.[5]

+ When portions are labeled *small*, people believe they are eating fewer calories regardless of the number of calories the foods contain or their actual size.[6]

+ When Oreo cookies are labeled as organic, people perceive them as having fewer calories than conventional Oreos. This happens even when the study subjects have been shown package labels indicating that calories are equal in both kinds of cookies.[7]

Studies suggest that *any* health label on a food product—"no trans fat," "vitamins added," "contains antioxidants," "contains probiotics"—will encourage customers to believe that the calories don't count, or don't count nearly as much.

THE DIETING EFFECT

Some research has suggested that overweight people tend to underestimate the number of calories they eat to a greater extent than do people of normal weight. It also suggests that the degree of underreporting increases with increasing overweight. But as Brian Wansink and his colleagues point out, underreporting is more likely to be due to the effect of the size of the meal than to weight itself. People who are overweight eat larger meals and, therefore, underestimate calories by a larger fraction. Although some studies suggest that people who are dieting deliberately underreport calorie intake, most research finds that nearly everyone underestimates calorie intake regardless of body weight or dieting status.[8]

THE "NEGATIVE CALORIE" (OR WISHFUL THINKING) EFFECT

We have argued throughout this book that calories do count, so we are especially amused by the claims of some diet books that certain foods use up more calories in digestion, absorption, and metabolism than they contained in the first place—that their thermic effects are greater than their calorie values. This, of course, is physiologically impossible. The maximum thermic effect of food, as we discussed in previous chapters, is 20 to 30 percent (for protein), which still leaves plenty of calories left over. The only example of negative calories that we can think of is what happens when you drink ice-cold water. Water has no calories, but it takes some heat—about 100 calories per quart—to warm it to body temperature. A quart is quite a lot of water, and ice-cold water is not always comfortable to drink. We do not view this method as a convenient way to waste calories.

But we enjoy negative-calorie studies, and here is a favorite. The investigator came up with the idea that "people intuitively believe that eating healthy foods in addition to unhealthy ones can decrease a meal's calorie count." To test this idea, he showed bowls of chili with and without a side salad to volunteers. On average, the study subjects guessed that the chili alone contained about 700 calories. But when they saw the chili along with a green salad, they thought the meal provided only 655 calories, 45 fewer than the chili alone—as if, as the investigator put it, the salad had negative calories. People who said they were dieting were twice as likely as nondieters to make this error.[9]

And then there are the claims of the Negative Calorie Diet, ostensibly "based on more than 100 negative calorie foods requiring your body to BURN more calories than the actual calorie content of the food itself!"[10] On this diet you are supposed to be able to eat all you want of more than a hundred negative-calorie foods, lose weight, and not feel hungry. What are these magic foods? Just the low-calorie, high-nutrient-density fruits and vegetables that you might expect to be recommended to someone who is dieting: celery, grapefruit, lemon, lime, apple, lettuce, broccoli, cabbage, and other such items. As Julie Upton explains in an article on myths about metabolism, "A medium-size rib of celery has only about 6 calories; its [thermic effect] is approximately half a calorie. In reality, 'negative calorie foods' are nothing more than wishful thinking."[11]

In practice, the negative-calorie idea fits well with the well-researched volumetric approach developed by Professor Barbara Rolls at Pennsylvania State University. Eating low-calorie fruits and vegetables helps with weight loss because they fill the stomach and make you feel satisfied.

THE "CALORIE OBLIVION" EFFECT

Overall, surveys and research studies consistently report widespread public misunderstanding of calories not only in food but also in the body. In May 2011, for example, the International Food Information Council, an educational arm of the food industry, published the results of its sixth annual survey of consumer attitudes toward food safety, nutrition, and health. The survey asked about perceptions of caloric intake and expenditure. Here are some of its findings:

+ Only 9 percent of respondents came close to estimating the correct number of calories they might need each day.
+ One-quarter thought they required 1,000 calories a day or less.
+ Sixty percent said they had no idea how many calories they needed to eat.[12]

These results were similar to those obtained a year earlier, when *USA Today* quoted the nutritionist Dawn Jackson Blatner: "Nobody knows how many calories they should be eating, nobody knows how many they are eating, and nobody knows how many calories are in foods. . . . I would say it's beyond calorie-confused. It's calorie-oblivious."[13]

Given widespread calorie oblivion, and short of doubly labeled water experiments, how are you supposed to know whether your calories are in balance? We know only one way: weigh yourself on a scale at regular intervals. If your calorie intake pretty much equals your expenditure, your weight should stay about the same over time, within a range of a couple of pounds. And your belt should not require adjustment.

But it is worth knowing about calorie oblivion for one other reason. The inability to judge calories with reasonable accuracy is reason enough to support better public education about calories in food and the number required to maintain body weight. And that brings us to recent efforts to improve calorie information on food labels and restaurant menus.

CHAPTER 23

Calorie Labeling
Science and Politics

One way to help people learn about calories is to list them on food labels, but mandatory calorie labeling is relatively recent in the United States. During much of the twentieth century the FDA officially allowed nutrition information on food labels only when food products were meant for the treatment of specific diseases or other "special dietary uses." We say *officially* because this restriction did not stop food companies from displaying information about added nutrients—and occasionally calories—when it helped to market their products. The FDA permitted them to do this as long as the labels did not display claims for health benefits.

Courtesy of the Kellogg Company, we have a complete collection of images of Rice Krispies cereal boxes dating back to 1928, the year the cereal was introduced. Rice Krispies labels did not display nutrients or calories until 1945, when the company began fortifying the cereal with added vitamins. Then as now, the calories in Rice Krispies derived from rice and added sugars.[1] Serving the cereal with milk increased the calories. The 1945 label lists 108 calories for a 1-ounce serving, but 186 with half a cup of whole milk. When Kellogg began to specify skim milk in 1985, the calories dropped to 150. Kellogg increased the serving size to 1.2 ounces in 1994, and current Rice Krispies labels list 130 calories per 1.2 ounces (170 with skim milk).

Cereal box labels reflect the history of nutrition labeling in the United States. Kellogg added vitamins to its cereals in response to reports of nutritional deficiencies among conscripts during World War II and the consequent demands of health authorities to fortify breads and other products made with refined flour. Despite this fortification, nutrient deficiencies remained entrenched in poverty areas of the United States. In 1969 the Nixon administration convened a White House conference aimed at ending hunger and undernutrition in the United States. Participants produced hundreds of recommendations, some of which led to the immediate expansion of federal food assistance programs.[2] Other suggestions, such as putting nutrition information on food labels, took longer to implement.

As we explain in chapter 25, the USDA is responsible for labels on meat and poultry products, and the FDA for those on most other foods. The FDA introduced new regulations for labeling foods under its jurisdiction in 1973. These rules made most labeling of nutrients voluntary. Nutrient labeling was mandatory only when manufacturers added vitamins or minerals to processed foods or claimed health benefits for their products. In such cases, the FDA required food companies to list the number of calories and amounts of nutrients per usual serving size.[3] Rice Krispies boxes had been listing nutrients as percentages of minimum daily requirements since the late 1940s, sometimes—but not always—with calories. As of 1974 they were required to list calories. They also had to list nutrients as percentages of Recommended Daily Allowances, as seen in figure 19.

Food manufacturers were well aware of the marketing potential of such listings and front-of-package messages about health benefits. In 1985 Kellogg filed a book-length petition with the FDA to allow health and nutrient-content claims on the front of food packages. Under pressure from food manufacturers and Congress, the FDA began developing mandatory regulations for the nutrition labeling of processed food products. Early in 1990 Dr. Louis W. Sullivan, the secretary of the FDA's parent agency, the Department of Health and Human Services, announced the rationale for these plans: "The grocery store has become a Tower of Babel, and consumers need to be linguists, scientists and mind readers to understand the many labels they see."[4]

Later that year Congress passed the Nutrition Labeling and Education Act (NLEA). This applied only to FDA-regulated foods and required the FDA to write the labeling regulations it was already writing. During the next few years the FDA wrote and rewrote labeling proposals in response to public comments. On January 6, 1993, the agency issued its final labeling

Kellogg's
RICE KRISPIES®

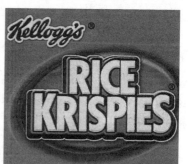

Kellogg's Rice Krispies is labeled in accordance with federal standards for nutrition labeling as established by the U.S. Food and Drug Administration.

These toasted puffs of rice are fortified with eight important vitamins and iron.

NUTRITION INFORMATION PER SERVING

SERVING SIZE: One ounce (1 cup) Rice Krispies alone and in combination with ½ cup vitamin D fortified whole milk.

SERVINGS PER CONTAINER: 13

	RICE KRISPIES	
	1 oz.	with ½ cup whole milk
CALORIES	110	190
PROTEIN	2 gm	6 gm
CARBOHYDRATES	25 gm	31 gm
FAT	0 gm	4 gm

PERCENTAGE OF U.S. RECOMMENDED DAILY ALLOWANCE (U.S. RDA)

	RICE KRISPIES	
	1 oz.	with ½ cup whole milk
PROTEIN	2	10
VITAMIN A	25	25
VITAMIN C	25	25
THIAMINE	25	25
RIBOFLAVIN	25	35
NIACIN	25	25
CALCIUM	*	15
IRON	10	10
VITAMIN D	10	25
VITAMIN B₆	25	25
FOLIC ACID	25	25
PHOSPHORUS	2	10
MAGNESIUM	2	6
ZINC	2	2

*Contains less than 2 percent of the U.S. RDA of these nutrients.

Nutrition Facts

Serving Size 1¼ Cups (33g/1.2 oz.)
Servings Per Container About 10

Amount Per Serving	Cereal	Cereal with ½ Cup Vitamins A&D Fat Free Milk
Calories	130	170
Calories from Fat	0	0

	% Daily Value**	
Total Fat 0g*	0%	0%
Saturated Fat 0g	0%	0%
Trans Fat 0g		
Cholesterol 0mg	0%	0%
Sodium 220mg	9%	12%
Potassium 30mg	1%	7%
Total Carbohydrate 29g	10%	12%
Dietary Fiber less than 1g	1%	1%
Sugars 4g		
Other Carbohydrate 25g		
Protein 2g		
Vitamin A	25%	30%
Vitamin C	25%	25%
Calcium	0%	15%
Iron	50%	50%
Vitamin D	10%	25%
Vitamin E	25%	25%
Thiamin	25%	30%
Riboflavin	25%	35%
Niacin	25%	25%
Vitamin B₆	25%	25%
Folic Acid	25%	25%
Vitamin B₁₂	25%	35%
Phosphorus	4%	15%

* Amount in cereal. One half cup of fat free milk contributes an additional 40 calories, 65mg sodium, 6g total carbohydrates (6g sugars), and 4g protein.

**Percent Daily Values are based on a 2,000 calorie diet. Your daily values may be higher or lower depending on your calorie needs:

	Calories	2,000	2,500
Total Fat	Less than	65g	80g
Saturated Fat	Less than	20g	25g
Cholesterol	Less than	300mg	300mg
Sodium	Less than	2,400mg	2,400mg
Potassium		3,500mg	3,500mg
Total Carbohydrate		300g	375g
Dietary Fiber		25g	30g

Calories per gram: Fat 9 • Carbohydrate 4 • Protein 4

FIGURE 19. Nutrition panels from boxes of Kellogg's Rice Krispies cereal from 1974 (above) and 2011 (right). The 1974 label follows FDA rules issued in 1973. The 2011 Nutrition Facts panel adheres to requirements of the Nutrition Labeling and Education Act of 1990 as implemented in 1994. These regulations were still in force in 2011. The 1974 label is courtesy of the Kellogg Company.

rules in a massive *Federal Register* notice of nearly 900 pages.[5] Those labeling regulations went into effect in 1994 and remain in place at the time of this writing, although the FDA has been working on the revisions we discuss in chapter 25.

CALORIES IN THE NUTRITION FACTS PANEL

In excruciating detail, the 1993 *Federal Register* notice specified elements of the Nutrition Facts panel—overall design, nutrient listings, font type and size, line width and length. The FDA based every decision about these details on its own research and on suggestions from the public and experts. Its final conclusions about the most seemingly trivial details—"Calories must be in a type size no smaller than 8 point"—were anything but random. Here we discuss the FDA's decisions about the display of calories, using the 2011 Rice Krispies panel in figure 19 (right panel) as an example.

The FDA's final rules required calories to appear in four places on the Nutrition Facts panel in four different ways: calories per serving, calories from fat, percent Daily Values, and Atwater Values. Public comments about calories were especially contentious. The FDA seriously considered listing energy in kilojoules as well as calories, in part because of complaints from scientists that *calories* was an outmoded term that got in the way of international trade and the exchange of scientific information. In rejecting this idea, the FDA noted that the law required it to use the most appropriate units on food labels. As a result, "the agency is not persuaded that the mandatory use of metric terminology, or the declaration of factors to convert calories to kilojoules, is justified."[6]

As noted in chapter 3, the FDA allowed manufacturers to calculate the number of calories in their products using any of five methods: (1) Atwater Values, (2) the USDA's 1955 Modified Atwater Values as slightly revised in 1973, (3) Atwater Values corrected for insoluble fiber, (4) calorie values approved by the FDA for specific foods, or (5) bomb calorimetry figures corrected for the loss of urinary nitrogen.[7] In deciding to allow such flexibility, the FDA recognized that the USDA's food composition tables had not been updated since 1955 and that current labels might underestimate calorie content. The agency was less concerned about overestimations, such as those obtained by bomb calorimetry, since those would not "be disadvantageous to the consumer."[8]

Calories per Serving

To list calories per serving, the FDA first had to define the sizes of standard servings—a monumental task. Using the amounts reported as consumed in dietary intake surveys, agency staff identified reference amounts commonly consumed (RACCs), or standard sizes, for 139 distinct food categories. Public arguments over the optimal sizes of RACC servings go on for pages in the 1993 *Federal Register*.

The FDA, for example, proposed a RACC for chocolate brownies of 40 grams, but the baking industry wanted it to be 80 grams, consistent with other cake servings. The FDA insisted on 40 grams because survey respondents said that was what they ate and the "FDA cannot change a reference amount simply to make it consistent with industry practice." Although it is impossible to know how accurately survey respondents reported their brownie consumption, the FDA stayed with the figures it had: "The reference amount must reflect the amount commonly consumed."[9]

Even in 1993, FDA serving sizes appeared small relative to what people actually ate. The serving size for ice cream, for example, is an ungenerous one-half cup, meaning that a pint contains an improbable four servings. Unlike bakers, most food manufacturers seemed satisfied with smaller serving sizes, not least because they make products appear to have fewer calories. If a pint of ice cream has 1,000 calories, a half-cup contains only 250.

Calories from Fat

The FDA developed the 1993 rules soon after the publication in the late 1980s of two major consensus reports on diet and chronic disease prevention, one from the government and one from the National Academy of Sciences. Both identified eating less fat—not fewer calories—as the top public health nutrition priority.[10] In response the FDA devoted considerable label space to amounts and types of fat. Because the reports advised restricting fat intake to no more than 30 to 35 percent of total daily calories, the FDA listed "calories from fat" to make the comparison easier. To allow for small errors, the agency said foods with fewer than 5 calories from fat could label them as 0. Foods containing up to 50 fat calories per serving had to be labeled to the nearest 5, and those with higher amounts had to be labeled to the nearest 10.

In the early 1990s health officials believed that reducing dietary fat intake would have two benefits. It would help people reduce calorie intake, because the calories in fat are more concentrated than those in protein or carbohydrate. And it would reduce saturated fat intake, because much of the fat in American diets comes from meat and dairy foods. It did not occur to the writers of these reports that the food industry would respond to the low-fat message by replacing the lost calories from fat with as many or more from sugars and starches—an approach that came to be known as the SnackWell phenomenon, named for Nabisco's wildly popular cookies that were made fat-free but by no means calorie-free.[11]

Percent Daily Value: 2,000-Calorie Diets**

The asterisks refer to a footnote, "** Percent Daily Values are based on a 2,000 calorie diet. Your daily values may be higher or lower depending on your calorie needs."

The FDA wanted consumers to be able to compare the amounts of saturated fat and sodium to the maximum amounts recommended for a day's intake—the Daily Values.[12] Because the allowable limits would vary according to the number of calories consumed, the FDA needed benchmarks for average calorie consumption, even though calorie requirements vary according to body size and other individual characteristics.

From USDA food consumption surveys of that era, the FDA knew that women typically reported consuming 1,600 to 2,200 calories a day, men 2,000 to 3,000, and children 1,800 to 2,500 (measured intakes, of course, might be higher). But stating ranges on food labels would take up too much space and did not seem particularly helpful. The FDA proposed using a single standard of daily calorie intake—2,350 calories per day, based on the average of USDA survey responses.[13] The agency requested public comments on this proposal and on alternative figures: 2,000, 2,300, and 2,400 calories per day.

Despite the now-observable fact that 2,350 calories per day is below the average requirements for either men or women obtained from doubly labeled water experiments, most of the people who responded to the comments judged the proposed benchmark as too high. Nutrition educators worried that it would encourage overconsumption, be irrelevant to women who consume fewer calories, and permit overstatement of acceptable levels of "eat less" nutrients such as saturated fat and sodium. Instead, they proposed 2,000 calories as:

+ consistent with widely used food plans
+ close to the calorie requirements for postmenopausal women, the population group most prone to weight gain

- ✦ a reasonably rounded-down value from 2,350 calories
- ✦ easier to use than 2,350 and, therefore, a better tool for nutrition education

Whether a rounding down of nearly 20 percent is reasonable or not, the FDA ultimately viewed these arguments as persuasive. It agreed that 2,000 calories per day would be more likely to make it clear that people needed to tailor dietary recommendations to their own diets. The FDA wanted people to understand that they must adjust calorie intake according to age, sex, activity, and life stage. It addressed the adjustment problem by requiring the percent Daily Value footnote on food labels for diets of 2,000 and 2,500 calories per day, the range of average values reported in dietary intake surveys.

Atwater Values

The last line of the Nutrition Facts panel sometimes gives the Atwater Values in calories per gram: fat 9, carbohydrate 4, protein 4. The FDA allows these figures to be included for educational purposes despite objections that the line takes up too much space and that hardly anyone knows how to use the information. Yet there they are, more than a century after Wilbur Atwater's death.

READING NUTRITION FACTS LABELS

As we peruse the 1993 *Federal Register* notice, it appears to us that the FDA was struggling to do the best it could with the information then available. Its staff tested public understanding of a variety of design options. The results showed that people had a great deal of difficulty understanding *any* of the proposed options. Faced with the need to get rules in place by the date specified by Congress, the FDA chose to use the "least worse" design, the best of a poorly understood lot. That the Nutrition Facts label is difficult to understand is a given. The FDA deals with label complexities by offering a lengthy Web-based guide to reading the panel, complete with test questions. Here is an example from its section on calories, including those from fat:

> There are 250 calories in one serving of this macaroni and cheese. How many calories from fat are there in ONE serving? Answer: 110 calories, which means almost half the calories in a single serving come from fat. What if you ate the whole package content? Then, you would consume two servings, or 500 calories, and 220 would come from fat.

TABLE 23 1993 FDA RULES FOR CALORIE-CONTENT CLAIMS

Calorie claim	FDA synonyms for calorie claim	Foods: calories per serving	Meals: calories per serving
Free	Calorie-free, zero-calorie, without, trivial source of, negligible source of, dietarily insignificant source of	Less than 5	As indicated by information on Nutrition Facts label
Low	Little, few, contains small amount of, low source of, low in	40 or less	120 or less per 100 grams
Reduced or Less	Lower, fewer	25 percent less than the regular food	25 percent less per 100 grams
Light	"Lite"	Food with 50 percent or more calories from fat: "lite" versions have 50 percent fewer fat calories Food with fewer than 50 percent calories from fat: lite versions have 33 percent fewer calories or 50 percent fewer fat calories	Must meet definition for low calorie or low fat

SOURCE: FDA, 1993 (see note 5).
NOTE: Claims can only be made when the product contains more than 40 calories per serving. When a food is naturally low calorie, the label may say, for example, "celery, a low-calorie food."

We suspect that most people would prefer not to have to bother with such calculations or to remember the General Guide to Calories given in that section: "40 Calories is low, 100 Calories is moderate, 400 Calories or more is high."[14]

NUTRIENT CONTENT CLAIMS: CALORIES

The 1993 *Federal Register* also listed rules for categories of health claims on food packages. One category, Nutrient Content claims, has rules for statements about calorie content.[15] These are so specific that we summarize them in table 23 on the previous page.

Food companies employ armies of lawyers to read and interpret such rules, and the FDA employs its own legions to write, enforce, and revise them. The need for revision has become increasingly urgent as rates of obesity, especially among children, continue to rise and elicit demands for better public education about diet and health in general and calories in particular. In the early 2000s the FDA began to examine the need for revising the food label. It had even more work to do when Congress passed health care reform legislation in 2010 that required calories to be posted on the menu boards of fast-food restaurants, which we discuss in chapter 25. But first let's take a look at the politics of nutrition labels on alcoholic beverages.

CHAPTER 24

Alcohol Labels

Industry vs. Consumers

Regulating alcohol, as we explained in chapter 11, is about tax revenues, not health. The end-of-Prohibition law passed in 1935 made the Treasury Department responsible for labeling hard liquor and most wines and beers. The department's Alcohol and Tobacco Tax and Trade Bureau (TTB) requires calories to be labeled only on beers marketed as *light*.[1] Other alcoholic beverages do not have to list calories, and most do not. If you want to know the number of calories in your drink, you can measure its volume and assume that standard servings of wine (5 ounces), light beer (12 ounces), and the hard stuff (1.5 ounces) have about 100 calories each. A 12-ounce regular beer has about 150. Larger volumes will have more, in proportion to their size.

The omission of calories on alcohol drink labels is not for lack of trying. Beginning in the early 1970s, the advocacy group Center for Science in the Public Interest (CSPI) spent more than twenty-five years unsuccessfully petitioning for more-informative labels.[2] At times during those years, variously named Treasury bureaus responded by proposing three kinds of labeling rules:

+ alcohol percent by volume, from which you can deduce calories
+ ingredients, some of which might provide calories
+ nutrition information, which, according to the TTB, means calories plus grams of carbohydrate, protein, and fat—nothing else

The history of efforts to regulate alcohol in the United States involved differing and sometimes surprising coalitions of advocates and lobbyists. It began in 1919 with Prohibition, the era following congressional ratification

TABLE 24   FEDERAL LABELING REQUIREMENTS FOR DISTILLED SPIRITS,
WINE, AND BEER

Beverage	Alcohol by volume	"Ingredients" (as defined by TTB): carbohydrate, protein, fat	Calories (nutrition information)
Distilled spirits	Yes (proof optional)	No, but permitted	No, but permitted*
Wine			
More than 14 percent alcohol	Yes	No, but permitted	No, but permitted*
7 to 14 percent alcohol	Yes, unless labeled *light* or *table*	No, but permitted	No, but permitted*
7 to 14 percent alcohol, light or table	No, but permitted	No, but permitted	No, but permitted*
Less than 7 percent alcohol (FDA regulated[†])	No, but permitted	Yes (Nutrition Facts)	Yes (Nutrition Facts)
Beer, malt beverage			
Regular	No, but permitted	No, but permitted	No, but permitted*
Light[† ‡]	No, but permitted	No, but permitted	Yes
Beer, nonmalt: (FDA regulated[†])	No, but permitted	Yes (Nutrition Facts)	Yes (Nutrition Facts)

*If labels disclose calories, they must also list grams of carbohydrate, protein, and fat.

[†]The FDA regulates wines containing less than 7 percent alcohol by volume and beers that are brewed from grains other than barley.

[‡]The alcohol content of light beer has no regulatory definition.

of the Eighteenth Amendment to the U.S. Constitution. This amendment prohibited the manufacture, transport, and sale of alcoholic beverages. Prohibition lasted from 1920 to 1933, when Congress repealed it by passing the Twenty-First Amendment. In 1935 Congress enacted the provisions of the Alcohol Administration Act, and these still apply.

The act established distinctly different rules for labeling wine, beer (specifically, malt beverages), and distilled spirits. No doubt for reasons having to do with revenue, its provisions apply only to wines containing at least 7 percent alcohol and to beers made from barley and hops that have been malted (sprouted) and fermented. The act excludes wines with less alcohol and beers made from any other fermented grain. The excluded products are regulated by the FDA, and inconsistencies abound.[3] We think the alcohol labeling rules are so peculiar that we summarize them in table 24. Although federal labeling requirements take precedent, the states are permitted to apply the regulations in different ways. They may, for example, set limits on alcohol content, the size of containers, or where and when alcoholic beverages may be sold—an unusual instance of state laws taking precedence over federal laws.

ALCOHOL CONTENT

If you know the percent alcohol of your drink, you can estimate its calories by plugging that value into the formula we gave in chapter 11. TTB regulations require the labels of hard liquor to state percent alcohol by volume. A statement of proof, which is twice the percent alcohol—80 proof whiskey is 40 percent alcohol, for example—is optional. The labeling rules for wines depend on how much alcohol they contain. Wines with more than 14 percent alcohol must state the percentage. Wines containing 7 to 14 percent alcohol must state the percentage unless they are labeled *light* or *table*. In contrast, products regulated by the FDA must display the usual Nutrition Facts panels and ingredient lists but do not have to disclose alcohol content.

The post-Prohibition Alcohol Administration Act explicitly prohibited beer labels from disclosing alcohol content: "The alcoholic content and the percentage and quantity of the original extract shall not be stated unless required by State law."[4] Regulators rightly believed that the disclosure of alcohol content would encourage beer companies to engage in alcohol wars, and they did not want beer to be marketed on the basis of alcohol strength.

In the late 1980s the Coors Brewing Company sued in federal court to overturn this labeling restriction. The company argued that the ban constituted an illegal restraint on free speech and violated the First Amendment. In 1991 a district court ruled in favor of Coors:

> The asserted government interest central to this case is the prevention of strength wars among the brewers.... It is a reasonable, legitimate legislative interest within Congress' commerce power ... to protect the consumer from the otherwise unchecked "mistakes and excesses" of the brewing industry.... [But] because the government has a relatively insubstantial interest in preventing strength wars when compared to the consumers' countervailing interest in disclosure, the statute is unconstitutional. In sum, we hold that Coors' proposal to advertise the alcohol content of beer is commercial speech protected by the First Amendment, and that the public's interests in disclosure are significant.[5]

The case went all the way to the Supreme Court, which upheld this ruling in 1995. Since then the TTB has permitted—but does not require—companies to label beer packages with alcohol content.[6] International beer brands in specialty stores tend to label alcohol content. But perhaps because the TTB forbids companies to market beer on the basis of strength, we find few domestic beers that label alcohol content, even those made by Coors. Domestic beers marketed as high-potency energy drinks seem to be an exception. In 2010 at a New York City drugstore, we found a Joose premium malt beverage that listed alcohol content—an impressive 9.9 percent—in *three* places on its label. That's one way to market strength.

INGREDIENTS

In 1972 CSPI petitioned the TTB's predecessor agency, then called the Bureau of Alcohol, Tobacco and Firearms (ATF), to require ingredient lists on alcohol labels. At the time CSPI was focused on exposing the potential hazards of food additives.[7] CSPI staff knew that alcoholic beverages contained artificial sweeteners, sulfites, and food dyes such as Yellow #5, to which some people are sensitive. For the next fourteen years CSPI continued to file petitions and sue the ATF to demand the labeling of additive as well as innate ingredients. In response the ATF went through cycles of denying petitions, proposing rules, responding to public comments, proposing more rules, and rescinding previous actions.

The ATF denied CSPI's petitions largely on the grounds that the costs to industry would outweigh the benefits to consumers. It did, however, recognize that the petitions had some merit and published rules for ingredient disclosure in 1980. Labels would not have to list ingredients if companies provided that information on request. They would not have to list ingredients in order of predominance or disclose those used in manufacture. Protective of industry as these rules may seem, the ATF rescinded them in 1981 when President Ronald Reagan insisted that federal agencies lessen the burden of federal regulations on business. In 1986 the courts supported the ATF's rationale for opposing ingredient labeling, concluding that the record "failed to establish that ingredient disclosure would provide useful information as to the actual contents of the alcohol beverage."[8]

In the early 1980s, the ATF required labels to disclose whether alcoholic beverages contain Yellow #5. It required disclosure of aspartame and sulfites in the early 1990s. But it did not—and does not—allow labels to list vitamins, minerals, or other nutrients or display health claims, lest manufacturers attempt to sell drinks on that basis. These policies are further complicated by the need to balance the extensive harm caused by the abuse of alcohol against the well-established benefits of moderate drinking for heart health. In *Food Politics*, Marion Nestle describes the furor over efforts by the wine industry to label bottles with a statement that "alcohol, in particular red wine, reduces the risk of heart disease."[9] To date, the TTB has denied requests to make such claims, but the industry keeps on trying.

We get some hints of more interesting ingredients when looking at FDA-regulated wines. A "strawberry white zinfandel" in our local wine store discloses white zinfandel, water, high fructose corn syrup [a calorie source], malt flavor, carbon dioxide, citric acid, potassium sorbate, potassium benzoate, and potassium metasulfate. It voluntarily discloses alcohol as 6 percent. With alcohol, corn syrup, and other carbohydrates, this drink contains 160 calories per 8-ounce serving.

But current Treasury regulations say nothing about ingredients in the 9.9 percent alcohol Joose "energy-boosting" beer we mentioned earlier, labeled as "with natural flavors, caffeine, ginseng, taurine, and FD&C Yellow #5 & 6." Whatever else these ingredients are supposed to do, they are not sources of calories. Late in 2010, as a result of several deaths among young people who had binged on such drinks, the FDA deemed caffeine unsafe to add to alcoholic beverages and blocked further sales of such products.[10]

NUTRITION INFORMATION: CALORIES

The only alcoholic beverages that are required to list calories are light beers and FDA-regulated wines and beers. For all others, calorie labeling is voluntary, which means hardly ever done, although Coors and some other companies disclose calories on their websites.[11] If such a label does display calories, it must also list the TTB's version of ingredients: carbohydrate, protein, and fat. But the protein and fat content of alcohol drinks is negligible, if not zero. Listing protein and fat serves little purpose except to distract from calories. The amount of carbohydrate in alcoholic beverages is also relatively small, ranging from less than 3 to a little more than 10 grams (two teaspoons) per standard serving.

In 1993 the ATF responded to a petition to require nutrition information similar to Nutrition Facts—but *not* ingredient lists—on alcohol labels.[12] Although it did not disclose the source of the petition, rumors pointed to

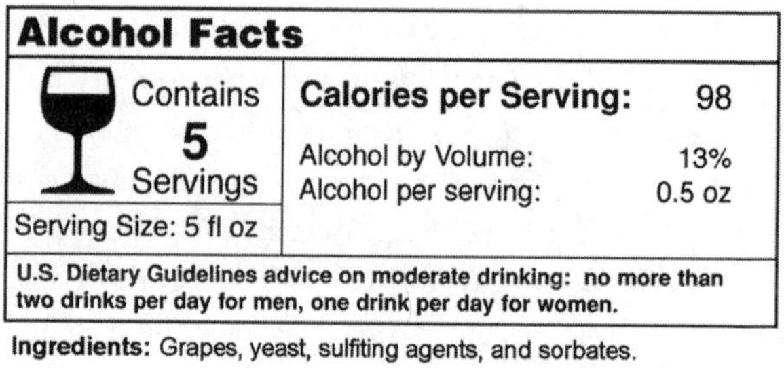

Alcohol Facts	
Contains **5** Servings Serving Size: 5 fl oz	**Calories per Serving:** 98 Alcohol by Volume: 13% Alcohol per serving: 0.5 oz

U.S. Dietary Guidelines advice on moderate drinking: no more than two drinks per day for men, one drink per day for women.

Ingredients: Grapes, yeast, sulfiting agents, and sorbates.

FIGURE 20. The Alcohol Facts label suggested by consumer groups. In 2003, consumer groups unsuccessfully petitioned the Treasury Department to require informative labels like this one for wine on all alcoholic beverages. Source: CSPI, 2003 (see note 14).

Diageo, the world's largest producer of distilled spirits. Government agencies were promoting low-fat diets in the early 1990s, and the makers of hard liquor thought it would help sales to label their products as zero fat. Because a standard 0.6-ounce serving of hard liquor provides only 100 calories, marketers could practically advertise these drinks as low-calorie, no-fat health foods.

The opposition to this creative marketing idea included strange bedfellows: the Wine and Beer Institutes but also CSPI, which did not want liquor companies marketing their products on the basis of nutritional value, let alone as diet foods. Given the almost universally negative reaction, the ATF concluded that there was no "convincing evidence that nutrition labeling would provide substantial useful information to consumers." It denied the petition, and stopped all rulemaking on the issue.[13]

Ten years later obesity had emerged as a major national health problem. CSPI joined with the National Consumers League and nearly seventy other consumer and health organizations to petition the agency, now called TTB, to require an Alcohol Facts panel on all beverages under its jurisdiction. The petitioners' proposed label listed alcohol by volume, serving size, alcohol per serving, calories per serving, ingredients, number of drinks per container, and a statement giving advice about moderate drinking for men and women, as shown in figure 20.

The petitioners argued, "Though many drinkers wish it were not the case, alcoholic beverages provide calories. Those calories may contribute to weight gain if consumed as part of a diet that provides more calories than a consumer expends. In addition, individuals who consume too many calories in the form of alcohol are at risk of malnutrition because they may be substituting alcohol

Serving Facts

Serving Size	12 fl oz (355 ml)
Servings Per Container	2

	Amt Per Serv.
Calories	90
Carbohydrate	2g
Fat	0g
Protein	1g

FIGURE 21. The TTB's 2007 proposed Serving Facts label for wines. The Serving Facts label does not have to display alcohol content as long as that information appears someplace on the package label. Source: TTB, 2007 (see note 18).

for more nutritious foods. . . . Providing calorie information on the labels of alcoholic beverages, as on foods and non-alcoholic beverages, is all the more important today, when obesity has become a national epidemic."[14]

The alcohol industry countered with its own petition, for *voluntary* labeling. The TTB supported the industry's approach, issued guidance about how to label products *voluntarily* with an optional Serving Facts—not Alcohol Facts—panel, and requested public comment on this proposal.[15]

But before the TTB announced these proposals, Diageo North America said that it planned to label its beverages with alcohol content and calories. The company could not wait to take advantage of the low-carbohydrate diet craze then under way. As one Diageo executive explained, "People have a lot of interest in carbohydrates, and wine has always been a low-carb beverage." At the time, one of us (Marion Nestle) commented, "They must think that having nutrition labels on alcoholic beverages might have a positive effect. . . . If they can get a consumer-friendly, healthy image on their products, they're going to do that."[16] Diageo placed an advertisement for Seagrams 7 in the April 20, 2005, *USA Today* displaying a Serving Facts label: "You can always count on 7. No fat, zero carbs and 97 calories per 1.5 ounce serving."

CSPI's response? "Simply stated, CSPI calls upon TTB to put the concerns of the public above the interests of alcohol producers, who seek labeling changes at least partly to enhance their competitive prospects and expand the market for their products. . . . Label declarations that tout the nutritive components of alcoholic beverages would obscure well-documented findings—and the consistent judgment of the Dietary Guidelines—that alcohol provides calories, but few essential nutrients."[17]

In 2007, after dealing with 19,000 comments on its proposals, most of them generated by Diageo, the TTB proposed new labeling rules. For the first time, these would be *mandatory*. Labels would have to list alcohol content and provide a Serving Facts panel, a watered-down version of CSPI's more informative Alcohol Facts. Lest even these requirements appear too onerous, companies would not have to state the alcohol content on the panel as long as it appeared someplace on the label.[18] Figure 21 (previous page) shows the alcohol-free version of the proposed Serving Facts label.

In January 2008 CSPI filed extensive comments on the proposal, quite sensibly insisting that the TTB reconsider the Serving Facts panel to make it list alcohol and ingredients but not the unnecessary fat and protein content. CSPI also demanded a dietary guidelines warning statement.[19] As of late 2011, the TTB has neither responded nor issued final rules. Its proposals apparently got caught in the 2010 midterm election cycle, and they remained in *Federal Register* limbo. CSPI, in a budget-cutting measure during the economic downturn in 2009, discontinued its Alcohol Policy Project.

In the meantime we see that the ever-innovative spirits industry has introduced a "thin-dustry" campaign to convince young women to link drinking liquor to weight loss. This campaign explains the popularity of the Skinnygirl margarita—"100 calories, . . . natural flavors, lightly sweetened with agave nectar . . . Skinnygirl is the margarita you can trust." It also explains Applebee's 100-calorie SkinnyBee margarita, which, the menu says, is "pretty cool when you realize you burn 3 calories just by lifting your glass to take a sip."[20] File this last marketing innovation under "calorie expenditure: wishful thinking."

CHAPTER 25

Will Calorie Labels Help Fight Obesity?

By the early 2000s federal health officials recognized that rates of obesity were rising rapidly, and they began looking for ways their various agencies could encourage individuals to take personal responsibility for controlling calorie intake. In this chapter we review U.S. efforts to educate the public about calories through better food labels and through city, state, and national laws requiring restaurants to post calorie information.

THE FDA'S LABELING REVISIONS

In 2003 the FDA created an internal Obesity Working Group (OWG) to assess how the agency might educate consumers about calorie balance. The OWG members, all FDA professional staff, were impressed by "the scientific fact that weight control is primarily a function of the balance of calories eaten and calories expended." They titled their report *Calories Count.*[1]

Calories Count dealt mainly with the legal restrictions on the FDA's food labeling regulations and the lack of research on public understanding of calories. The OWG urged the FDA to develop design options for revising the food label, conduct research to find out how well the options were understood, and base revisions on the results of that research. This was not something the FDA could do quickly. The agency is legally required to announce its rulemaking intentions, open proposals for public comment, respond to the comments, propose rules, open them for comment, and respond to these comments. Only then can it issue final rules. FDA processes require interminable *Federal Register* notices and proceed at glacial speed (pre–global warming). The FDA kicked off the new labeling initiative in 2005 with requests for comments about how it could help improve public understanding of calorie labels and encourage consumers to choose smaller portion sizes.[2]

Calories Count argued that food labels should give less attention to fat and more to calories. Following the scientific low-fat consensus of the late 1980s, food companies replaced fat calories with carbohydrate calories. In the ensuing decade Americans increased their calorie intake from all sources. Obesity, the OWG said, was a result of overconsumption of calories from any source, not just fat. The OWG advised the FDA to require listing calories on the front of food packages in clear, bold lettering. It also advised labeling a package likely to be consumed by one person at one sitting as if it were a single serving. The label for a 20-ounce soft drink, for example, would have to disclose 275 calories for the bottle rather than 110 for 1 serving (and 2.5 servings).

The FDA conducted focus groups to test consumer views of the single-serving idea and identified much confusion about multiple servings per package. But its request for comments came out in 2005, during the antiregulatory years of the Bush II administration, and labeling revisions came to a halt. After the administration changed in 2009, the FDA announced that it intended to be more active in labeling matters. Anticipating that the agency would soon get around to proposing regulations, Coca-Cola and PepsiCo voluntarily began to list total calories and calories per serving on the Nutrition Facts labels of soft drinks containing up to 20 ounces. In February 2011 they and other soda companies proudly announced that drinks up to that size would display the total number of calories on the *front* of the container. Larger bottles, however, would continue to display calories per serving.[3]

FDA'S LABEL RESEARCH PROJECTS

Soft drink companies were correct in assuming that the new FDA administration was serious about revising food labels. In 2009, the FDA began the long, slow process of updating the Nutrition Facts panel. And for the first time, it took an active interest in front-of-package marketing symbols that had been proliferating on food packages. The agency intended to develop a uniform nutrition ranking system to replace them. The FDA was particularly concerned about consumer understanding of the way the Nutrition Facts panel conveyed information about calories, serving sizes, and Daily Values.

It announced that its researchers would be soliciting responses from several thousand participants to a variety of formats through a Web-based interview process. The results of its studies were expected to be released late in 2011. The agency also announced that it would be addressing the confusion caused by the plethora of symbols and check marks developed by food companies, health organizations, and other private groups to indicate self-designated "better-for-you" products. It wanted to replace these with a uniform symbol that would be easy for consumers to notice and use. Although many of the labeling schemes displayed calories, their value to the public was unclear.[4]

To address some of these concerns the FDA recruited the Institute of Medicine (IOM) to evaluate the strengths and weaknesses of about twenty front-of-package labeling schemes. The IOM issued its first report in 2010. It recommended that only four items be included in front-of-package labels, those considered to be overconsumed by Americans: calories, saturated fat, trans fat, and sodium. Note the surprising absence of sugars. The committee chose not to list sugars or total fat because, it said, calories took care of both. The IOM's second committee took care of the sugar gap. Based on the Dietary Guidelines released in 2010, the IOM told the FDA it should adopt a system that included sugars. The committee recommended a uniform front-of-package symbol system that would display calories per serving but also rate foods on their content of three elements: solid fats (saturated and trans), sodium, and sugars.[5]

How the FDA will respond to this report remains to be seen. As for the research, FDA scientists presented their preliminary findings on public understanding of front-of-package design options late in 2010. Consumers, they found, were better able to identify healthier options from nutrient-based labels (e.g., red, yellow, and green traffic lights) than summary labels (check marks). None of the options, however, "inspire[d] consumers to focus on nutrition when making product decisions."[6] How could they? We cannot imagine how one front-of-package symbol could possibly summarize a food's individual contribution to calorie balance, nutrient density, and calorie density.

THE USDA'S FOOD LABEL INITIATIVES

The nutrition labeling law passed by Congress in 1990 applied to foods regulated by the FDA, not the USDA. For reasons dating back to the original food safety laws of 1906, Congress split food regulation between the two agencies, making the USDA responsible for meat and poultry and the FDA responsible for pretty much everything else. Although the USDA did not have to, in 1991 it proposed mandatory nutrition labeling requirements comparable to the FDA's, but only for multi-ingredient and heat-processed meat and poultry products. It announced the final rules for these products on the same day that the FDA issued its rules for Nutrition Facts labels, in January 1993.[7]

For all other meat and poultry products, the USDA made nutrition labeling voluntary. The voluntary categories included raw products and those produced by small businesses, enclosed in small packages, or packaged at the retail level. In 2001, when USDA officials realized that most meat producers were not using nutrition labels voluntarily, they proposed mandatory rules. That proposal languished during the Bush II administration. The Obama USDA revived the proposal in 2009 and issued final rules at the end of 2010. These require producers to put the USDA's version of Nutrition Facts labels on most packaged raw meat and poultry, whether intact or ground, by January 1, 2012.[8] Figure 22 gives an example.

As shown in the figure, a 4-ounce serving of this "90 percent lean" ground meat contains 11 grams of fat and 21 grams of protein. But 52 percent of its 190 calories come from fat. The greater the fat content, the higher the calories. A fattier "75 percent lean" ground beef provides 320 calories per serving from 28 grams of fat and 18 grams of protein. Meat producers much prefer to label their products by percent lean than percent fat.

Meat producers also want to promote the value of their products as sources of protein. Unlike FDA labels, USDA labels establish a Daily Value for protein of 50 grams per day. FDA labels list grams of protein but not as a percent of Daily Value, because Americans typically consume more than twice the amount of protein required in daily diets. This particular product provides 41 percent of the protein Daily Value in just 4 uncooked ounces. Saying so makes meat appear exceptionally nutritious and also distracts from its content of saturated fat and calories. The industry has long opposed putting Nutrition Facts labels on meat, and we assume that the unnecessary Daily Value for protein must have been part of a compromise effort to get meat producers to go along with the new requirements.

In requiring these labels by 2012, the USDA brought its current policies in line with the rules the FDA had implemented nearly two decades earlier. New FDA label revisions will again leave the USDA behind. Chalk this up to meat industry pressures to reveal as little as possible about the calories, fat,

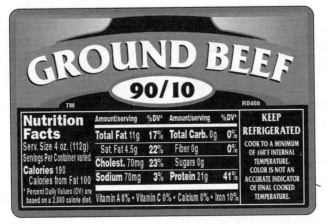

FIGURE 22. A USDA-regulated Nutrition Facts label for ground beef. This product is 90 percent lean and 10 percent fat by weight. USDA labels list calories per uncooked 4-ounce serving. They differ from FDA Nutrition Facts labels in several minor and one major detail: the display of a Daily Value for protein.

and saturated fat in its products and to the absurdity of dividing the regulation of one food supply between two agencies.

CALORIES ON RESTAURANT MENUS

When the Nutrition Labeling Act of 1990 went into effect in 1994, it specifically exempted restaurants from its regulations. The health care reform act of 2010 removed that exemption. Buried on page 455 of that 906-page law is "Nutrition Labeling of Standard Menu Items at Chain Restaurants," a section requiring chains with 20 or more units nationwide to post calories "in a clear and conspicuous manner" along with "a succinct statement concerning suggested daily calorie intake." These restaurants must disclose calories on menus and menu boards, next to self-service items, and on vending machines.[9]

Let's credit the Center for Science in the Public Interest (CSPI) for this one. In 2003 this venerable food and nutrition advocacy organization issued a report arguing that information about calories in restaurant meals would help people eat more healthfully. The report summarized the kinds of evidence we reviewed in chapter 21: more people eat meals away from home than ever before, children consume twice as many calories at restaurants as they do at home, and nearly everyone underestimates the calorie content of restaurant meals.[10] The FDA's Obesity Working Group picked up on CSPI's idea about calorie labeling in its 2004 *Calories Count* report when it recommended point-of-sale nutrition information in restaurants. The FDA asked the Keystone Center, a nonprofit group devoted to conflict resolution on matters of public policy, to conduct meetings of representatives from industry, government, academia, and the public sector to review the status of such information. The Keystone Center submitted its report to the FDA in 2006. It said that although about half of the chains that it surveyed provided calorie information, most put it in places where it was unlikely to be seen (on the bottom of McDonald's tray liners, for example). The report recommended more accessible calorie posting and further research to discover how this information might affect restaurants and their customers.[11]

By all accounts the public was highly interested in seeing calorie information. Some preliminary studies suggested that menu labeling might lead to reductions in purchased calories, particularly when accompanied by a statement referring the number in specific foods to a diet of 2,000 calories a day. But other early studies reported no effect or suggested that labeling might encourage people to eat more calories, especially young men (who seem especially susceptible to "strength" promotions). Because these studies were mostly done in laboratory settings and used indirect measures of food consumption, their real-life significance was unclear.[12]

New York was the first city to require calorie labels on restaurant menus. In 2006 the NYC Health Department proposed requiring quick-service chain restaurants with more than fifteen units within city limits to post calories on menu boards. The New York Restaurant Association strongly opposed this idea, arguing that calorie labeling would be impractical, expensive, and an unconstitutional violation of free commercial speech. It filed lawsuits. After much legal wrangling, the courts ruled in favor of the city, and menu labeling went into effect on July 19, 2008.[13]

Such strong opposition demonstrated that restaurants were unlikely to post calories voluntarily. Yet by 2009, California, Oregon, and Maine required calorie labeling, as did a dozen or more counties and cities. At least thirty other jurisdictions were considering similar bills. Confronted with a cacophony of differing laws that would present chains with difficult compliance problems, the Restaurant Association dropped its opposition. This paved the way for the national legislation that preempted local and state laws. While we waited for the national law to go into effect, the NYC experience provided an opportunity to find out whether menu labels would improve purchases, teach the public about calories, or induce restaurants to reduce the calories in their foods. Seeing the first calorie postings in 2008 gave us a severe case of sticker shock. We were stopped cold to discover that a large but quite thin chocolate cookie at Pain Quotidien weighed in at 670 calories.

Researchers went right to work to evaluate the effects of menu labeling. The early results of their first, short-term studies have been mixed, with most reporting limited or no effects on consumer behavior. Later NYC Health Department surveys also had mixed results. On average, they found little decline in purchase of calories. Some chains experienced declines but others did not. Most customers said they did not use the calorie information. But a key finding was that customers who did use the information were more likely to choose lower-calorie items.[14] Once national menu labeling is fully implemented, it will take several more years before its effects are known.

Whether menu labeling will convince restaurants to reformulate their products is also uncertain. From our collection of nutrition brochures obtained from fast-food outlets before and after NYC's menu labeling initiative, we can discern no clear trend. Some chains seem to have decreased calories by small amounts, but others have introduced new supersize items loaded with calories. The NYC Health Department found some chains to have reduced the calories in their menu items by 5 to 15 percent.[15]

If our personal observations of calorie postings are typical, restaurants are dealing with the New York law with considerable foot dragging. Some post calories in numbers too small or obscure to read easily. Others post to the absurdly precise single calorie—497 for a sandwich at the Cosi chain, for example. Some provide calorie information only if we ask for it. Those that allow customers to choose their portions tend to post calories in unhelpful ranges: 170–780 for a Chipotle salad, or 330–890 for ice cream at Cold Stone Creamery. And one comparison of actual measurements to the posted amounts found wide deviations, sometimes by as much as twofold.[16]

The FDA tackled such issues when it began to write the regulations for national menu labeling. It began by requesting information about present practices. Later it issued guidance to help restaurants comply with the forthcoming regulations. The guidance document addressed some of the foot dragging. It specified type styles and sizes and required rounding off to the nearest 5 or 10 calories, depending on the total. But it allowed restaurants to pick numbers based on "nutrient databases, cookbooks, laboratory analyses or other reasonable means." Early in 2011 the FDA withdrew the guidance and began the lengthy formal rulemaking process by opening the proposed labeling rules for public comment. The rules devote considerable attention to the problem of calorie ranges, which the FDA proposes allowing. They omit any mention of posting calories for drinks containing alcohol, although some chain restaurants serve such drinks. These drinks, of course, contain calories not only from the alcohol itself but also from juices, whipped cream, and other caloric mixers. This omission was sure to be a major topic of public comment. While waiting for those comments, the FDA told restaurants to start posting calorie information right away.[17]

ARE CALORIE LABELS WORTH THE TROUBLE?

Given the logistic problems and the limited evidence of benefit to date, it is worth considering the educational value of calorie labels. Their purpose is to promote personal responsibility for informed food choices. Calories, as we have explained repeatedly, are otherwise abstract; they cannot be seen, smelled, or tasted, and their biological functions are difficult for most people to grasp. Almost everyone underestimates calories in away-from-home foods, especially when portions are large or promoted as healthful. Explaining how food choices fit into a 2,000-calorie diet could help. So could explicit illustration that larger portions have more calories. That the calories in McDonald's french fries increase from 230 (small) to 380 (medium) to 500 (large) should be instructive to anyone who pays attention. We think menu labels and referral to 2,000-calorie diets can be useful educational starting points.

But we recognize that not everyone pays attention and that the early research results show that posting calories is useful for only a small percentage of customers at fast-food chains. Food choices, as we have repeatedly emphasized, are only partially about personal responsibility. Mostly they are about biological imperatives to defend body weight in the context of an "eat more" food environment. That is why some critics of calorie labeling are concerned that it might do more harm than good, not least because it might "substitute for, or delay, more substantive policies that get at the root of the problem."[18] Although we strongly support calorie labeling on restaurant menus, we believe that more effort should focus on ways to improve the food environment to make it easier for people to make healthier choices, as we discuss next, in our concluding chapter.

Conclusion

How to Cope with the Calorie Environment

We said at the outset that *Why Calories Count* is not a dieting or weight loss book. Instead, we wrote it to equip you with tools you might find useful for evaluating diet claims and developing your own weight management strategies for gaining or losing or just staying where you are. From our review of the research, we are convinced that calories count. If you want to lose weight, you really do need to eat less and move more than you have been doing. But let's be clear: you must also eat *better*, which means making healthier food choices.

If your reaction to these words is to yawn or groan, we are right with you. This is old news. It is also advice that ignores how hard it is for mere mortals to maintain or lose weight in an "eat more" food environment. In theory, biology regulates food intake within rather narrow limits. But in practice the food environment tests those limits. Biological regulatory mechanisms may fail miserably when constantly confronted with appealing food in large quantities. Genetics has plenty to do with weight regulation, but the presence of overabundant food, marketed aggressively and, sometimes, deceptively, profoundly distorts its effects.

If, like most people, you do not notice how food marketing affects your food choices, it is because you are not supposed to. You are especially not supposed to notice how it affects your children. If you want to eat less, eat better, and be more active, you must—on your own—find strategies for coping with "eat more" pressures from food marketers and your own biology.

Arguments about coping strategies invariably center on questions of responsibility. Are you solely responsible for your own or your family's food choices? Or do the food industry and government have some role? We think all are involved. If you view gaining weight as a matter of personal responsibility, you may blame yourself—or others—for an inability to control calorie intake. You may overlook the need to develop strategies to deal with biological and marketing pressures to eat more.

You do not make food choices in a vacuum. You select your diet on the basis of what's available, what you can afford, what's marketed, and what your friends are eating, as much as—or even more than—what you think might be good for you. We hope this book encourages you to pay much more attention to food marketing and its effects. You cannot change your own biology. But you can find ways to counter environmental pressures to eat more food, more often, and in larger amounts.

Here we suggest several strategies, recognizing that some will be easier to follow than others. We see nothing wrong with starting with the easy ones. These sometimes can make a big difference. Our plan has five steps: Get organized. Eat less. Eat better. Move more. Get political.

GET ORGANIZED

Once you realize that maintaining or losing weight opposes strong biological and environmental "eat more" forces, you can systematically explore ways to counter them.

Get Motivated

It helps to have a good reason for dealing with calorie imbalance. Whether that reason is health, appearance, pleasing someone who is worried about your weight—or outrage at food industry marketing pressures—use it to motivate action. Managing weight and eating better make many people feel better. Feeling better is reason enough. Go for it.

Monitor Your Weight

The best way to track calorie balance is to monitor your weight. Successful dieters buy a scale and weigh themselves regularly. If pounds creep up, they eat more carefully. Weight normally fluctuates by a few pounds from day to day as a result of water balance. Food is mostly water, and water is heavy—

16 fluid ounces to a pound. The amount of salt also matters, as it tends to retain water in the body. If you eat carbohydrates, some will be stored as glycogen, which binds four times its weight in water.

Don't worry about daily fluctuations of a pound or two, but do watch for longer-term trends. It is much easier to take off one or two pounds than five, ten, or more. You can now find electronic scales on the market that give instantaneous readings of weight, BMI, and body fat content and transmit the results to an Internet application that plots the data and creates your personal record of day-to-day weight fluctuations. If you enjoy tracking data, such scales can be fun to use. But regular use of any scale has been shown to improve the success of weight loss regimens.[1]

If You Like Groups, Join One

Many people find it easier to lose or maintain weight with social support. Weight loss groups and commercial diet plans offer structured ways to lose a few pounds. Without recommending particular plans, we can say we prefer the ones that emphasize variety, allow you to eat foods you like, and do not restrict entire categories of nutrients or foods. Point-counting systems, for example, assign a few or zero points to fruits and vegetables but loads of points to sodas and desserts. The points correspond to nutrient values as well as calories.

EAT LESS

If you have been gaining weight, you are eating more calories than you are expending. To stop the weight gain, you must reverse that trend. If you often eat at restaurants, this will be especially difficult, and you must watch out for a few extra "eat more" pitfalls.

Be Aware of Calories, but Don't Count Them Obsessively

This advice may seem surprising coming from us. We do think everyone should have a ballpark idea of calorie needs and the calories in foods, which is why we favor food and menu calorie labels. But we can't advise calorie counting as a weight loss strategy, because it is too difficult to do precisely. Unless you weigh everything you eat and know how the foods were prepared, your guess is likely to be too far off to be helpful. Weight Watchers calls this the calorie delusion and instead suggests using its point-counting system. If you don't want to bother with points, it might be just as easy to eat less (smaller portions, less frequently), eat better (healthier foods), and weigh yourself regularly.

Pick a Diet That Works for You

We think the most effective diet is one that helps you eat less and eat better in whatever way you most enjoy. Popular diet plans do the "eat less" part either overtly or covertly:

- *Low fat:* restricts calories from meat, full-fat dairy, and fried foods
- *Low carbohydrate:* restricts calories from bread, potatoes, pasta, desserts, and sodas
- *Low glycemic index:* restricts calories from foods containing rapidly absorbable sugars and starches
- *Vegetarian, vegan:* restricts calories from meat and dairy foods
- *No food mixing:* restricts calories from one or another food group
- *Volumetric:* requires eating more low-calorie fruits and vegetables

If these diets help you cut down on calories, you ought to lose weight while following them. Some fit into the "eat better" category more than others. If you already eat a varied diet of foods you like, find a way to eat less of them. Whatever you do, try to make changes you will be able to live with for the long term.

Insist on Smaller Portions

If there is one message to take home from this book, it is this: larger portions have more calories. Large portions alone are enough to upset your calorie balance. They are most often a problem when eating out, especially because the goal of restaurants is to get you to eat more, not less. Some restaurants may offer half-size portions (at 80 percent of the price, of course), but we find this approach to be rare. You can insist on ordering an appetizer instead of an entrée, immediately cut your entrée in half and save the rest to take home, share the entrée with friends, or order half portions when available (and see figure 23 for an additional suggestion). Bakery items are especially challenging, as they are often big enough to share with three or four friends. Try this: friends don't let friends eat whole portions.

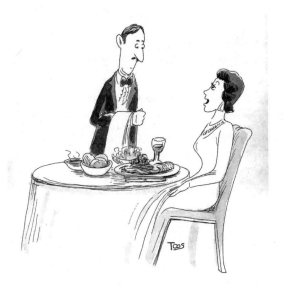

"I'll pay double for half as much."

FIGURE 23. Why won't restaurants serve smaller portions?
Some consumers will try anything to get them to, counter-
intuitive as this particular approach may seem. Andrew Toos,
www.CartoonStock.com.

Keep Snacks to a Minimum

Some people control their weight better if they eat frequent small meals throughout the day. Not us, alas. From where we stand, if eating large portions is the single best way to add calories to a diet, snacking comes in a close second. If you, like us, have problems with snacking, consider making some personal rules about where and when to eat. If you can't resist eating junk foods, don't have them in the house. We like keeping nuts, fresh fruit, and raisins in the house as snacks, but we are easily satisfied with small handfuls. Candy, however, is a problem. If it is at hand, we eat it. We only buy it occasionally, and in small amounts.

If you like to snack, try coming up with some healthier options. Sometimes just cutting up fruits and vegetables is enough to make them easier to eat, especially for kids. Read food labels. And watch out for power bars: they are marketed for their health aura but are not calorie-free (we view them as marginally better-for-you candy bars).

Eat What You Like

Food is about pleasure as well as calories. That is why we have said not a word about low-calorie food items, although we happen to like skim milk and low-fat yogurt. With those exceptions, we greatly prefer eating real foods and find them more satisfying than the diet alternatives. We like sugar too much to replace it with anything as chemical tasting as artificial sweeteners, and the mere idea of going on a low-carbohydrate diet is too depressing to contemplate. Give up bread and pasta? Not a chance. But we are lucky enough to be able to stop when we've had enough. If you can't do that—and we know many people who can't—choosing foods with a low glycemic index (those low in rapidly absorbable sugars and starches) is always a good idea, as is setting some limits on the size and frequency of desserts and sugary drinks. Everything is fine in moderation. But if you can't do moderation, you had best figure out some limits you can live with.

EAT BETTER

Yes, this book is about calories, but we must say it again: nutritional health is about much more. The nutrients in foods matter to health as much as calories do. While it is certainly possible to lose weight eating nothing but fast food and Twinkies, we do not recommend that approach. Diet makes a difference to health, and it is worth making it a habit—the default—to eat healthfully while balancing calories. For the last time, we invoke Wilbur Atwater, this time for his 1894 advice that American food habits could be greatly improved by eating less *and* eating better:

> Taking the results as they are, they very decidedly confirm the general impression of hygienists that our diet is one-sided and that we eat too much. The food which we actually eat, leaving out of account that which we throw away, has relatively too little protein and too much fat, starch, and sugar. This is due partly to our large consumption of sugar and partly to our use of such large quantities of fat. . . . How much harm is done to health by our one-sided and excessive diet no one can say. Physicians tell us that it is very great.[2]

Don't Drink Your Calories

For many people, especially kids, the best way to reduce calories is to cut down on sugary drinks. With nothing but "empty" calories, sodas have a

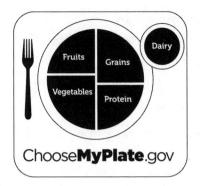

FIGURE 24. The USDA's 2011 food icon and guide. This icon, which replaces the 2005 MyPyramid food guide, is linked to specific suggestions about how to balance calories by eating less and eating better. From the USDA's MyPlate at www.choosemyplate.gov.

nutrient density of zero. Think of them, as the Center for Science in the Public Interest does, as liquid candy.[3] You would not let your child eat candy all day long, and the same should go for sodas. Try water.

Follow Dietary Guidelines

Despite public impressions that dietary advice changes all the time, the opposite is true. In the decades that we have been teaching and writing about nutrition, basic dietary advice has consistently promoted the same principles:

- ✦ Balance calorie intake with expenditure.
- ✦ Eat more fruits, vegetables, and whole grains.
- ✦ Eat less meat and dairy (and choose low-fat options).
- ✦ Eat less of junk foods high in calories from fats and sugars.[4]

The 2011 edition of the USDA's food guide says much the same thing, beginning with, "Enjoy your food, but eat less," as we show in figure 24.[5] As we have said from the start, eating better involves eating more foods of high nutrient density—lots of nutrients relative to calories. It also favors foods of low calorie density—few calories for the weight of the food. Fruits, vegetables, whole grains, fish, lean meats, and low-fat dairy products are foods of relatively high nutrient density *and* low calorie density. Junk foods are not.

Stay Out of Supermarket Center Aisles

Junk foods take up huge proportions of supermarket real estate, as Marion Nestle describes in her book *What to Eat*. If you must set foot in those aisles, she offers several suggestions, some only slightly facetious. Avoid food products with:

+ more than five ingredients (too highly processed)
+ ingredients you can't pronounce (bad-tasting chemical additives)
+ artificial ingredients (they taste bad and can never be tested enough)
+ a cartoon on the package ("eat more" marketing directed at kids)[6]
+ a health claim on the package (these are inherently deceptive)

Yes, these admonitions are exaggerated—healthy exceptions exist—but they should help you identify packaged junk foods that are best reserved for special treats and occasions rather than consumed as everyday fare.

MOVE MORE

Current guidelines for physical activity say that adults should engage in moderately intense activities for more than two hours per week and do something that strengthens muscles about twice a week. This can seem daunting if you don't like going to gyms, as we do not. But *moderate* means any brisk action: walking, gardening, dancing, bicycling, and many other enjoyable activities. And it doesn't have to be done all at once. The CDC says that ten minutes of walking three times a day adds up to the weekly goal.[7] The overall principles are encouraging: more activity is better than less, and some is better than none. Start with some. Then add more when you are ready.

Fidget

We are impressed by studies showing large differences in calorie expenditure based on fidgeting behavior. Try standing when using a computer, getting up frequently to walk around, and pacing around the back of the room at meetings. We like the "instant recess" approach proposed by Dr. Toni Yancey, a professor at UCLA. She suggests taking ten-minute exercise breaks at four-hour intervals throughout the day.[8] If that seems like too much, start with five minutes.

Turn Off the TV

Watching TV, researchers said in 1985, might actually cause obesity. When you watch TV, you are most likely to be sitting or lying down, bombarded by commercials for junk foods, watching programs with junk foods embedded in the content, and munching on advertised products. In 2010, children and adolescents spent an average of nearly eight hours a day using sedentary

TABLE 25   "GET POLITICAL" STRATEGIES TO SUPPORT "EAT LESS, EAT BETTER, MOVE MORE"

Goal: Healthier food environments

Public education
Improve calorie labels
Expand calorie labels on restaurant menus
Restrict misleading health claims on food packages
Provide clear, unambiguous dietary advice
Provide nutrition education in schools
Provide cooking instruction as needed

For children
Restrict food advertising and marketing aimed at children
Make healthy kids' meals the default
Make school meals universal
Provide healthier school lunches
Get vending machines and junk foods out of schools
Teach kids to grow food
Teach kids to cook

For adults
Ask restaurants to provide incentives for ordering smaller portions and provide
    incentives to restaurants for doing so
Provide insurance incentives for healthier diet and activity patterns
Develop pricing incentives to buy fruits and vegetables
Provide access in inner cities to farmers' markets and stores selling fruits and vegetables

---

Goal: Healthier activity environments

For children
Establish sidewalks and bike paths
Develop walk-to-school programs
Reintroduce school physical education
Establish safe places to play

For adults
Create bike lanes on city streets
Open stairwells in buildings
Establish workplace "instant recess" programs
Create automobile-free zones in cities

Goal: Healthier political environments

Promote gardens, local farms, and farmers' markets
End unhealthful agricultural subsidies
Tax soft drinks
Democratize election campaign contribution laws to blunt excessive corporate influence
    on food policy
Regulate Wall Street pressures on corporations to grow rapidly

---

SOURCE: Adapted from Nestle and Jacobson, 2000 (see note 10).

media, primarily television but also computers, video games, and devices for listening to music. The average U.S. adult spends hours more in such sedentary pursuits. Researchers have demonstrated consistently over the years that the amount of time spent watching TV predicts obesity and the conditions for which obesity is a risk factor.[9]

GET POLITICAL

Personal responsibility as we see it also means working to change the food environment to make it easier for everyone to eat less, eat better, and move more. The food environment is what sociologists like to call *socially constructed*, meaning that people made it the way it is. It is not inevitable. It can be changed. Your biology may be fixed, but you can do plenty to improve the environment in which biology operates.

In table 25 (previous page) we summarize policy actions that target changing the food environment.[10] These actions aim to make food, activity, and political environments healthier for people and the planet. All of these draw on grassroots political democracy to make meaningful changes. Singly no one of these changes is likely to reverse obesity trends, but together they could make a powerful difference.

From this collection of suggestions—get organized, eat less, eat better, move more, get political—we advise picking, choosing, and experimenting to find strategies that work for you. We particularly commend the "get political" actions to your attention. Become part of the local, sustainable, healthy food movement that has attracted so many of your neighbors who want to eat more healthful diets while supporting local farmers, strengthening communities, protecting soil and water, and discouraging climate change. It's not enough to "vote with your fork." It is also necessary to vote with your vote. Working to change the political system from the bottom up will help achieve a food environment that encourages food corporations to act more ethically and permits elected officials to represent public—rather than corporate—interests.[11] This is democracy in action at its best.

Overall, we love eating too much to deprive ourselves of the pleasures of the table or suggest that anyone else do so. If you also love to eat, you will want to find ways to make it easier for you and everyone else to eat the calories you enjoy—in moderation, of course.

Selected Events in the History of Calories, 1614–1919

1614	Santorio Sanctorius publishes the first metabolic balance studies relating food to body weight and excretions.[1]
1668	John Mayow publishes tracts on how flames require air and muscle action also requires "combustible matter."
1757	Joseph Black identifies carbon dioxide formed during respiration.
1762	Albrecht von Haller announces the mechanical theory of metabolism.
1772	Carl W. Scheele discovers oxygen but delays publishing his findings.
1774	Joseph Priestly publishes his independent discovery of oxygen.
1775	Antoine Lavoisier also discovers oxygen independently, recognizes it as an element, and names it.
1779	Adair Crawford publishes his experiments on animal heat.
1783	Lavoisier and Pierre-Simon Laplace construct a whole-body animal calorimeter to study the metabolism of guinea pigs.
1789	Lavoisier relates oxygen uptake to human energy metabolism, relates oxygen to combustion in and out of the animal body, and uses the terms *calorimeter* and *caloric*.
1795	George Pearson analyzes the chemical composition of potatoes.
1824	In lectures, Nicolas Clément defines *calorie* as a unit of heat and distinguishes large from small calories.
1827	William Prout classifies food components as saccharine (carbohydrate), oily (fat), and albuminous (protein).
1836	François Magendie separates foods into proteins, fats, and carbohydrates.

1840	Germain Hess determines that energy changes involved in chemical reactions are independent of where they take place; "burning" sugar in the body or in a flame produces the same amount of heat (Hess's law).
1842	Justus Liebig publishes his text on animal metabolism. Julius R. Mayer relates heat to mechanical work.
1843	Charles Chossat systematically studies the effects of starvation in pigeons.
1846–48	Julius R. Mayer publishes papers discussing definitions of *kilogram-calorie*, or *Calorie*.
1847	James Joule determines the mechanical equivalent of heat.
1848	James Henry Salisbury publishes his prize essay on the chemical composition of Pennsylvania corn.
1849	H. V. Regnault and J. Reiset devise a closed system for respiration studies and measure the relationship between oxygen consumed and carbon dioxide excreted (later known as the Respiratory Quotient, or RQ).
1852	P. A. Favre and J. T. Silbermann define *calorie*. Physics textbooks use *Calorie* as a unit of work.
1862	Max von Pettenkofer and Carl von Voit build a calorimeter large enough to measure oxygen consumption and carbon dioxide output in humans.
1864	W. Henneberg and F. Stohmann develop calorimetric and chemical methods to analyze the composition of foods.
1866	Von Voit conducts studies of calorie balance in humans and defines calorie requirements. Edward Frankland measures the heats of combustion of common foods.
1878	Joule uses *calorie* as a unit of heat.
1879–81	Marcellin Berthelot describes a bomb calorimeter, defines *Calorie*, and distinguishes a gram-calorie from a kilogram-Calorie by capitalizing a letter.
1882	Werner von Siemens proposes *joule* as a unit of electrical energy.
1885	Max Rubner demonstrates that heat produced per unit of body surface area is the same for all warm-blooded animals, defines heat in gram-calories, demonstrates that the energy laws of physics apply to caloric balance, and determines energy values for carbohydrates (4.1 calories/gram), fats (9.3), and proteins (4.1).
1887	Wilbur O. Atwater publishes articles about the potential energy of food in *Century*.
1888	The British Association for the Advancement of Science uses *joule* to define the energy requirements of work and introduces *Therm* to indicate heat energy (discarded in 1896).

1891   E. H. Jenkins and A. L. Winton compile analyses of American feedstuffs, demonstrating the value of food composition data.

1892   Atwater and E. B. Rosa begin the construction of a respiration calorimeter to measure human heat exchange.

1893   Adolf Magnus-Levy uses a portable respiratory exchange device to measure metabolic rates in hospitalized patients.

1894   Atwater publishes *Foods: Nutritive Value and Cost.*

1896   Atwater and A. P. Bryant publish *The Chemical Composition of American Food Materials*, giving fuel values per pound based on Rubner's values.

1897   Atwater and C. F. Langworthy publish their summary of more than 3,600 studies of nitrogen, carbon, and energy balance.

1899   Atwater and Bryant determine caloric values for protein (4 per gram), fat (8.9), and carbohydrate (4) in more than 4,000 foods.

1902   Henry Armsby performs his first experiments at Pennsylvania State College with a respiration calorimeter large enough to house cows. Atwater and Alfred C. True publish *Principles of Nutrition and Nutritive Value of Food.*

1903   Atwater designs his own bomb calorimeter.

1904   Atwater and Francis Benedict build a whole-body calorimeter to measure human energy intake and expenditure.

1907   Benedict begins his studies of calorimetry and energy metabolism. Atwater dies.

1909   *The New Century Dictionary* defines *kilocalory.*

1918   Lulu Hunt Peters publishes the first calorie-counting diet book in America, *Diet and Health with Key to the Calories.*

The Respiratory Quotient (RQ)

As we explained in chapter 4, measurements of energy expenditure, either through oxygen uptake or, as in the case of doubly labeled water, carbon dioxide output, must be corrected for the fuel—the mix of proteins, fats, and carbohydrates—that is being metabolized. The correction factor is called the respiratory quotient (RQ). It is the ratio of exhaled carbon dioxide to oxygen inhaled and metabolized. In chemical notation, this ratio is expressed as CO_2/O_2.

THE RQ (CO_2/O_2) FOR GLUCOSE

The complete oxidation of 1 mole (the molecular weight in grams) of the sugar glucose uses 6 moles of oxygen and yields 6 moles of exhaled carbon dioxide $(6CO_2/6O_2)$ plus 673 calories (this is a measured value). Because the ratio of exhaled carbon dioxide to inhaled oxygen is 6 divided by 6, the RQ for glucose is 1. The reaction is:

Glucose + 6 oxygen → 6 carbon dioxide + 6 water + 673 calories

In chemical notation, this is:

$$C_6H_{12}O_6 + 6O_2 \rightarrow 6CO_2 + 6H_2O \text{ plus 673 calories}$$

One more point: 1 mole of either oxygen or carbon dioxide has a volume of 22.4 liters. Therefore, for glucose the energy equivalent of 1 liter of oxygen

is 673 calories divided by 6 moles of oxygen times 22.4 liters/mole (673 / [6 ×
22.4]), which equals 5.0 calories. Similarly, the energy equivalent of 1 liter of
carbon dioxide exhaled is 5.0 calories.

THE RQ FOR FAT

The equation for the oxidation of a typical fatty acid, in this case palmitic
acid (16 carbons, no double bonds), is:

Palmitic acid + 23 oxygen → 16 carbon dioxide + 16 water + 2,392 calories

Fat is indeed highly caloric. In chemical notation:

$$C_{16}H_{32}O_2 + 23O_2 \rightarrow 16CO_2 + 16H_2O + 2,392 \text{ calories}$$

In this instance the RQ is $16CO_2/23O_2$, or 0.7.

For this particular fatty acid the energy equivalent of a liter of oxygen is
2,392 divided by 23 × 22.4, which gives 4.6 calories, and for a liter of carbon
dioxide exhaled it is 6.7 calories.

But the average value for fats containing a mixture of fatty acids is closer
to 4.7 calories per liter of oxygen. Since all food fats are mixtures of different
kinds of fatty acids, fats are considered to produce 4.7 calories per liter of
oxygen inhaled and used.

THE RQ FOR PROTEIN

Food and human proteins are made up of 20 different amino acids. These are
oxidized through a number of biochemical pathways. A representative protein is considered to have an RQ of about 0.83 and to produce about 4.7 calories per liter of oxygen and 5.6 calories per liter of carbon dioxide.[1]

THE RQ FROM MIXED DIETS

The RQ—the ratio of carbon dioxide to oxygen—varies with the fuel source,
as shown in table 26. The other columns in the table give calories per liter of
oxygen and Atwater Values to help clarify the differences between the various ways of counting calories.

But people do not eat pure fuels; they eat foods that contain mixtures

TABLE 26   RESPIRATORY QUOTIENTS, CALORIES PER
LITER OF OXYGEN, AND ATWATER VALUES FOR PROTEIN,
FAT, AND CARBOHYDRATE: SUMMARY

Food component	Respiratory quotient, CO_2/O_2	Calories per liter of oxygen	Atwater Values, calories per gram
Protein	0.83	4.7	4
Fat	0.7	4.7	9
Carbohydrate	1.0	5.0	4

of protein, fat, and carbohydrate. The RQ depends on that mix but also on how recently food was consumed. Among people who have just eaten, the RQ is usually close to 1, indicating that carbohydrate is preferentially being metabolized for energy.[2] In people who have been fasting for many hours, however, the RQ is usually closer to 0.7 because metabolism draws on stored fat as a source of energy (see chapter 13). For times in between, the RQ gives some idea of the mix of fuels undergoing metabolism.

Frequently Asked Questions

We wrote *Why Calories Count* to answer the many questions that we had about this subject and thought others might have. Knowing that we were working on this book, friends and colleagues asked many more. We tackled most of them in the relevant chapters, but others seemed enough off-topic or so specific to weight loss that we preferred to address them in an FAQ.

Does cooking foods increase their calories?

Sometimes yes, sometimes no. This idea is the basis of a book by the anthropologist Richard Wrangham, *Catching Fire: How Cooking Made Us Human*. Civilization, Wrangham says, became possible once humans began to cook their food. Cooking reduces the energy cost of digestion, leaving more energy available for brain development. Perhaps so, but as we discussed in chapter 5, the energy cost of digestion is quite small—less than 1 percent of the original calories in foods. What cooking does is to improve the digestibility of some plant foods, especially tubers; it makes their calories more accessible so fewer of them are excreted. Cooking particularly improves the digestibility of raw potato starch and also destroys some enzyme inhibitors and plant toxins in other foods. But raw meats are digested as well as cooked meats, and the starch in many uncooked legumes and cereals is efficiently digested. And some anthropologists say that the taming of fire came much later in human evolution than the development of large brains.[1]

Does eating slowly help reduce calorie intake?

It might, though not by much. In theory, it ought to take some time for regulatory factors to be secreted and do their work, and some research supports this idea. But tests of the speed question have to be controlled for amounts consumed. For example, Japanese researchers compared the weights of men and women who said they ate quickly or slowly, but also whether they ate until full or not. Rates of overweight were twice as high among people who said they ate quickly until full as compared to people who reported eating slowly until full or not full. But the slow eaters were not eating as much. As for satiety, U.S. researchers report that slow eaters consume fewer calories and feel more satisfied than fast eaters. A Dutch study found slow eating to be associated with a small but not statistically significant decline in measured calorie intake.[2] If there is a difference, it seems small. But you can give slow eating a try and see if it works for you. Tell impatient dinner partners that eating slowly is part of your weight maintenance strategy.

How about chewing food for a long time? Will that help me eat less?

Shades of Horace Fletcher! We thought the peculiar fad invented by the Great Masticator went out with Lulu Peters almost a century ago (see chapter 18), but no such luck. Nutritionists in Harbin, China, recently counted the number of times obese and lean people chewed their food: the lean subjects chewed their foods longer. The investigators assigned subjects to chew foods either 15 or 40 times before swallowing. The result? The 40-chew groups took in 12 percent fewer calories and displayed lower levels of the "eat more" signal ghrelin and higher levels of the "stop eating" signal cholecystokinin (see table 16 in chapter 12). The investigators concluded, "Interventions for improving chewing activity could become a valuable adjunctive tool for combating obesity."[3] Maybe, if the tedium keeps chewers from overeating (the calories expended in chewing, alas, are trivial). We have our doubts about long-term efficacy, not least because practitioners will drive their dinner partners crazy, but hope Mr. Fletcher is smiling in his grave.

Does eating breakfast help you maintain weight?

Successful dieters enrolled in the National Weight Control Registry report eating breakfast every day, along with monitoring body weight and exercising frequently. This observation suggests that eating breakfast might be a useful weight loss strategy. But while some reports say that eating breakfast is satiating and reduces overall calorie intake, others find just the opposite—eating just a little or even skipping breakfast is a good way to *reduce* calorie intake.[4] Our advice? Do what works best for you.

Can you really lose six pounds in two weeks eating Special K breakfast cereal?

Maybe, if you follow its hilarious diet plan. You are to eat one "sensible" meal a day and replace the other two with Special K cereal or other Kellogg diet products. You also are allowed two Kellogg diet snack products a day—and fruit and vegetables as additional snacks.[5] If your one meal really is sensible and you don't eat too much cereal, you probably won't be eating many calories. Depending on how big your calorie deficit turns out to be, you will lose weight. We don't think this diet sounds like a reasonable long-term strategy (for anyone except Kellogg), but it ought to work for any dieter willing to stick to it for a couple of weeks.

Will frequent snacking help you lose weight?

Investigators at Pennsylvania State University tested the effects of yogurt snacks on the amount of food consumed at a buffet lunch. Participants ate less at lunch if they had eaten the yogurt within the previous half hour. But if they ate the yogurt any earlier, they did not eat less lunch, and whether the yogurt was high in fat or carbohydrate made no difference. In this and other studies, the calories from snacks were not compensated for by eating less at the next meal, an observation that supports the idea that the more often you eat, the more calories you are likely to consume.[6]

Can I really burn 300 calories in 15 minutes?

Maybe *you* can. We can't. We've seen such claims on the covers of women's magazines. But if you weigh 130 pounds, jumping rope or running upstairs nonstop for 15 minutes will burn only 150 to 200 calories (see chapter 8). You would have to do something much more vigorous to burn 300 calories in 15 minutes.

Will eating fast food make you gain weight?

It depends on how much you eat, obviously. But fast food often gets blamed for rising rates of obesity, and for good reason. Fast food has a high energy density—a large number of calories relative to the weight of the food. Foods high in fat, sugars, and processed starches but low in fiber are energy dense. Some research shows that humans tend to eat about the same weight of food every day, regardless of the number of calories. If this is true, eating foods of high energy density will lead you to eat more calories. Such foods are thought to overwhelm the physiological controls of the appetite. In *The End of Overeating*, David Kessler notes that fast food is deliberately engineered to please people's taste preferences so they will want to eat more of it. Morgan Spurlock, in his film *Super Size Me!*, gained twenty-five pounds in a month from eating all his meals at McDonald's. But other people have lost weight by eating only at McDonald's because they kept their calorie intake below expenditure.[7]

Do overweight people gain weight more quickly than so-called normal-weight people?

No, they do not. The number of calories needed to gain weight depends on the initial body weight and body fat content. Once people are overweight, they seem to deposit a larger proportion of excess calories as fat than do lean individuals. Fat tissue takes more excess calories to deposit—it stores more calories—than lean tissues. Overweight people must eat more calories than lean people to increase their body fat stores and gain weight.[8]

Will weight loss drugs help me lose weight?

Maybe, but the side effects may not be worth it. Pharmaceutical companies love the idea of diet drugs, as the market for them is enormous and people would have to take them for life. As we suggested in chapter 12, finding a drug that controls weight is a challenge. To date, such drugs produce only modest weight loss, and the weight usually comes right back when drug therapy stops. In the United States most drugs once thought to be promising have been removed from the market or denied approval because of the harm observed from long-term use. Those that remain are prescription drugs approved for use in obese patients at high medical risk. Such drugs can be used for up to twelve weeks in patients with BMIs above 30 (or above 27 in patients with a concurrent obesity-related condition).[9] Potential side effects preclude longer-term use.

Only one anti-obesity drug is presently approved for long-term use in the United States: orlistat, marketed as Xenical or Alli. This drug inhibits the enzyme that digests fat in the intestine. When taken with a meal, it reduces fat digestion by about 30 percent, thereby reducing calorie intake. The undigested fat passes to the large intestine, where it can cause flatulence, fecal urgency, oily stools, and anal leakage.[10] These symptoms are so unpleasant that takers quickly learn to eat low-fat diets to minimize symptoms—a strategy that can also reduce calorie intake.

As for efficacy: one clinical trial gave orlistat to obese patients with type 2 diabetes. After four years, 52 percent of the patients taking orlistat—*and* eating a reduced-calorie diet—completed the study and maintained an average weight loss of 7 percent. But only 34 percent of people taking a placebo completed the study; they had an average 4 percent weight loss after four years.[11] The 3 percent difference is either impressive or not, depending on how desperate you are. And you still need to eat a reduced-calorie diet to achieve weight loss. But because almost any weight loss is associated with improved glucose tolerance, obesity specialists consider orlistat an effective treatment.

What about surgery?

The purpose of obesity ("bariatric") surgery is to force patients to reduce their calorie intake by reducing their stomach capacity. More than 100,000 such surgeries are done in the United States each year. One procedure creates a small stomach pouch and isolates it from the remaining stomach. Another places an adjustable band around the stomach to create a small pouch that empties into the remaining stomach. These procedures make it difficult to eat more food (and therefore calories) than the small pouch can hold and they require substantial changes in eating behavior. They may influence appetite, perhaps by affecting intestinal hormones. Bariatric surgery can result in substantial weight loss—50 pounds or more—that can be maintained over many years. Studies show that for severely obese individuals, the surgery can improve risk factors for diabetes and cardiovascular disease and reduce overall mortality. But like any surgery, this one has a downside. The complication rate is on the order of 8 percent and consequences can be severe. For that reason the American Diabetes Association cautions that bariatric surgery should be considered only for people with a BMI of 35 or more who have failed to respond to other therapies. It says the evidence is insufficient to recommend the surgery to people with lower BMIs unless they are enrolled in a research study. Because of the hazards and the need for lifelong medical monitoring and support, we and others view surgery as a last resort for people trying to balance calories and lose weight.[12]

Is it true that calories don't count if you eat:

- *desserts that are hot (the calories burn off)?*
- *foods that are less than one inch in diameter (e.g., chocolate kisses, cheese cubes)?*
- *diet soda (it cancels out calories in foods)?*
- *at a movie or any other place of entertainment?*
- *in a car, airplane, or any other form of transportation?*
- *off someone else's plate (those are their calories)?*
- *where nobody sees you?*
- *foods sold for charity (these get a religious dispensation)?*
- *standing up (something to do with gravity)?*
- *in front of the TV (something to do with radiation)?*
- *foods on toothpicks (something to do with leakage)?*
- *foods intended for children (they must have fewer calories)?*
- *foods that don't taste good?*
- *foods with writing on them (e.g., "Happy Birthday")?*
- *foods that would otherwise be thrown away?*

Alas, these are all wishful thinking and classic myths about calories.[13] Not one of them is true, but we like them anyway.

NOTES

ABBREVIATIONS

AJCN   *American Journal of Clinical Nutrition*

Am   *American*

ATF   Bureau of Alcohol, Tobacco, Firearms and Explosives (until 2003, Bureau of Alcohol, Tobacco and Firearms)

Bull   Bulletin

CDC   Centers for Disease Control and Prevention

CSPI   Center for Science in the Public Interest

FAO   Food and Agriculture Organization of the United Nations

FDA   U.S. Food and Drug Administration

FR   *Federal Register*

GAO   Government Accountability Office (until 2004, General Accounting Office)

HHS   U.S. Department of Health and Human Services

Int'l   *International*

IOM   Institute of Medicine of the National Academies

J   *Journal, Journal of, Journal of the*

JADA   *Journal of the American Dietetic Association*

JAMA   *Journal of the American Medical Association*

NEJM   *New England Journal of Medicine*

NYT   *New York Times*

Res   *Research*

Suppl   Supplement

TTB   Alcohol and Tobacco Tax and Trade Bureau

U   University, University of

USDA   U.S. Department of Agriculture

WHO   World Health Organization of the United Nations

WSJ   *Wall Street Journal*

INTRODUCTION

1. Olshansky SJ, et al. A potential decline in life expectancy in the United States in the 21st century. *NEJM* 2005;352:1138–45.

2. Brownell K, Horgon KB. *Food Fight: The Inside Story of the Food Industry, America's Obesity Crisis, and What We Can Do about It.* New York: McGraw-Hill, 2004.

3. Nestle M, Nesheim MC. *Feed Your Pet Right.* New York: Free Press / Simon and Schuster, 2010.

4. Nestle M. *Food Politics: How the Food Industry Influences Nutrition and Health,* revised edition. Berkeley: U California Press, 2007.

5. Wansink B. *Mindless Eating: Why We Eat More than We Think.* New York: Bantam, 2010.

1. WHAT IS A CALORIE?

1. Hargrove JL. Does the history of food energy units suggest a solution to "calorie confusion"? *Nutrition J* 2007;6:44 at www.nutritionj.com/content/6/1/44.

2. Code of Federal Regulations. Title 21. Section 104-20(d).

3. FDA. Food labeling: Mandatory status of nutrition labeling and nutrient content revision, format for nutrition label: Final rule. *FR* 1993;58:2082.

2. THE HISTORY: FROM ANCIENT GREECE TO MODERN CALORIE SCIENCE

1. Jouanna J. *Hippocrates* (DeBevoise MB, tr). Baltimore: Johns Hopkins U Press, 1999.

2. *Hippocrates* (Jones WHS, tr), Vol. IV. Loeb Classical Library. Cambridge, MA: Harvard U Press, 1931:383.

3. Lusk G. *Clio Medica X. Nutrition.* New York: Paul B. Hoeber, 1933:8. The Hippocrates aphorism and quotation are from *Hippocrates* (Jones WHS, tr), Vol. IV, 1931:105, and Vol. VI, 1931:367.

4. Hippocrates (Jones WHS, tr), Vol. IV, 1931:333. Galen. *On the Parts of Medicine; On Cohesive Causes; On Regimen in Acute Diseases in Accordance with the Theories of Hippocrates* (Lyons M, tr). Berlin: Akademie Verlag, 1969:110,85–86.

5. Lusk G, 1933:26. The figure is from Quincy J. *Medicina Statica: Being the Aphorisms of Sanctorius* [William Newton, 1718]. London: Wellcome Library.

6. Carpenter KJ. A short history of nutritional science: Part 1 (1785–1885). *J Nutrition* 2003;133:638–45.

7. Kleiber M. *The Fire of Life: An Introduction to Animal Energetics.* New York: John Wiley and Sons, 1961. Kleiber, a University of California animal nutritionist, paid tribute to Lavoisier's contributions in this influential book. Its title recognizes the role of oxygen in both flames and metabolism.

8. Hargrove JL. History of the calorie in nutrition. *J Nutrition* 2006;136:2957–61. Zeigler MR. The history of the calorie in nutrition. *Scientific Monthly* 1922;6:520–26.

9. Carpenter KJ. The life and times of W.O. Atwater (1844–1907). *J Nutrition* 1994;1707s–14s.

10. Atwater WO. The potential energy of food. The chemistry and economy of food. III. *Century* 1887;34:397–405. Quotation: 403.

11. Atwater WO. *Foods: Nutritive Value and Cost.* USDA Farmers' Bull No. 23, 1894:9.

12. Atwater WO, Langworthy CF. *A Digest of Metabolism Experiments in Which the Balance of Income and Outgo Was Determined.* USDA, 1897. Quotations: 7, 9.

13. True AC. Letter of transmittal. In: Atwater WO, Woods CD. *Dietary Studies with Reference to the Food of the Negro in Alabama in 1895 and 1896.* Washington, DC: USDA, 1897:3.

14. Mudry JJ. *Measured Meals: Nutrition in America.* Albany: SUNY Press, 2009:39, 171, 175.

15. Cullather N. The foreign policy of the calorie. *Am Historical Review* 2007;122:337–64. Cullather N. *The Hungry World: America's Cold War Battle against Poverty in Asia.* Cambridge, MA: Harvard U Press, 2010. This thoughtful book deals with how Green Revolution agricultural development efforts in Asia in the 1960s affected Western attempts to stop the spread of Communism during the Cold War.

3. FOODS: HOW SCIENTISTS COUNT THE CALORIES

1. McMurry J, Fay RC. *Chemistry,* 4th ed. Upper Saddle River, NJ: Prentice Hall, 2003, figure 8.9.

2. Rubner's table is reproduced in Atwater WO. The potential energy of food. The chemistry and economy of food. III. *Century* 1887;34:401.

3. Atwater WO, Bryant AP. The availability and fuel value of food materials. *Twelfth Annual Report of the Storrs Agricultural Experiment Station,* 1899. Middletown, CT: Storrs Agricultural Experiment Station, 1900:73–110.

4. Atwater WO. *Principles of Nutrition and Nutritive Value of Food.* USDA Farmers' Bull 142 (2nd rev), 1910. Cited in: Merrill AL, Watt BK. *Energy Value of Foods . . . Basis and Derivation.* USDA Agricultural Handbook No. 74, February 1973. Although Atwater is listed as the author of the 1910 report, he died in 1907.

5. Maynard LA. The Atwater system of calculating the caloric value of diets. *J Nutrition* 1944;28:443–52.

6. Merrill AL, Watt BK. *Energy Value of Foods . . . Basis and Derivation*. USDA Agricultural Handbook No. 74, March 1955. The 1973 edition says it was "Slightly revised, February 1973."

7. Merrill and Watt (previous note) state that the diet includes Japanese persimmons (1,834 g), peanuts (213 g), tomatoes (11 g), a whole-wheat product called granose (28 g), olive oil (7 g), and milk (57 g).

8. Allison RG, Senti FR. *A Perspective on the Application of the Atwater System of Food Energy Assessment*. Bethesda, MD: Life Science Research Office, Federation of American Societies for Experimental Biology, 1983:iv.

9. Code of Federal Regulations. Title 21: Food and Drugs, Part 101—Food Labeling, Section 101.9, Nutrition Labeling of Food, available at www.accessdata .fda.gov/scripts/cdrh/cfdocs/cfCFR/CFRSearch.cfm?fr=101.9.

4. BODIES: HOW SCIENTISTS MEASURE THE USE OF CALORIES

1. It takes 80 calories (as we use the term) to melt a kilogram of ice.

2. Atwater WO, Woods CD, Benedict FG. *Report of Preliminary Investigations on the Metabolism of Nitrogen and Carbon in the Human Organism, with a Respiration Calorimeter of Special Construction*. Washington, DC: USDA Office of Experiment Stations, 1897:34.

3. See Pennsylvania State University Alumni Association, Historical Marker Guide, Index of Markers, http://alumni2.psu.edu/VRPennState/HistMrkr/Index. html, under "Calorimeter."

4. Benzinger TH, et al. Human calorimetry by means of the gradient principle. *J Applied Physiology* 1958;12:s1–s28.

5. Rumpler WV, et al. Repeatability of 24-h energy expenditure measurements in humans by indirect calorimetry. *AJCN* 1990;51:147–52. Baylor College of Medicine. Children's Nutrition Research Center. Lab—Energy metabolism, at www.bcm .edu/cnrc/index.cfm?pmid=9610.

6. Even in the late nineteenth and early twentieth centuries, scientists had chemical methods for measuring the amount of oxygen in air. Today they have machines for analyzing oxygen.

7. Kleiber M. *The Fire of Life: An Introduction to Animal Energetics*. New York: John Wiley and Sons, 1961:125.

8. Lifson NR, McClintock R. Theory of use of the turnover rates of body water for measuring energy and material balance. *J Theoretical Biology* 1966;12:46–74. Schoeller DA. Measurement of energy expenditure in free-living humans by using doubly labeled water. *J Nutrition* 1988;118:1278–89.

9. Schoeller DA, et al. Energy expenditure by doubly labeled water: Validation in humans and proposed calculation. *Am J Physiology* 1986;250:R823–30.

10. Schoeller DA. Human energy metabolism: What have we learned from the doubly labeled water method? *Annual Review of Nutrition* 1991;11:355–73. IOM. *Dietary Reference Intakes for Energy*. Washington, DC: National Academies Press, 2005:164–222.

5. METABOLISM: HOW THE BODY TURNS FOOD INTO ENERGY

1. Carnivores and herbivores process foods differently depending on the way their stomachs are organized and where microbial fermentation takes place. But once proteins, fats, and carbohydrates enter the small intestine, digestive enzymes process these molecules the same way in all species.

2. When proteins escape digestive enzymes and are somehow absorbed into the body, they can induce allergies or prion diseases. Pandeya DR, Acharya NK, Hong S-T. The prion and its potentiality. *Biomedical Res* 2010;21(2):111–25.

3. Mitchell HH, Hamilton TS, Beadles JR. The nutritional effects of heat on food proteins with particular reference to commercial processing and home cooking. *J Nutrition* 1949;39:413–25. Fleming SE, Vose JR. Digestibility of raw and cooked starches from legume seeds using the laboratory rat. *J Nutrition* 1979;109:2067–75.

4. The energy trapped during the conversion of ADP to ATP amounts to about 7,300 calories per mole of ATP. This seems like a great deal of energy, but one mole of ATP (or anything else) contains 6×10^{23} molecules.

6. THE FIRST USE OF CALORIES: BASIC LIFE FUNCTIONS

1. Lusk G. *Nutrition*. New York: Paul B. Hoeber, 1933:117.

2. Mitchell HH. *Comparative Nutrition of Man and Domestic Animals*. New York: Academic Press, 1962:3.

3. Woo R, Daniels-Kush R, Horton ES. The regulation of energy balance. *Annual Reviews of Nutrition* 1985;5:411–33. IOM. *Dietary Reference Intakes for Energy*. Washington, DC: National Academies Press, 2002.

4. Kleiber M. Body size and metabolism. *Hilgardia* 1932;6:315–53.

5. Harris JA, Benedict FG. *A Biometric Study of Basal Metabolism in Man*. Carnegie Institution of Washington, Publication 279, 1919. The formula for men: BMR (heat/24 hours) = 66.4730 + (13.7516 × body weight in kg) + (5.0033 × height in cm) − (6.7550 × age in years). For women: BMR = 655.0955 + (9.5634 × body weight in kg) + (1.8486 × height in cm) − (4.6756 × age in years).

6. FAO. *Human Energy Requirements*. Report of a joint FAO/WHO/UNU expert consultation, Rome, 17–24 October 2001:Annex 3.

7. Schofield WN. Predicting basal metabolic rate, new standards, and review of previous work. *Human Nutrition, Clinical Nutrition* 1985;39(suppl 1):5s–41s. For men ages 30 to 60, for example, the BMR = (11.3 × weight in kg) + (16 × height in m) + 901. For women ages 30 to 60, the BMR = (8.7 × weight in kg) − (25 × height in m) +

8[65]. The formulas differ for men and women in three other age groups: 10–18, 18–30, and >60 years. See WHO. *Energy and Protein Requirements*, 1985:Annex 1 (online at FAO, Corporate Document Repository at http://www.fao.org/DOCREP/003/AA040E/AA040E00.HTM).

8. BMR calculator at www.bmi-calculator.net/bmr-calculator. This calculator and most others online are based on Harris-Benedict equations.

9. Gallagher DD, et al. Organ tissue mass measurement allows modeling of REE and metabolically active tissue mass. *Am J Physiology—Endocrinology and Metabolism* 1998;275:E249–58.

7. THE SECOND USE: HEAT LOSSES WHILE METABOLIZING FOOD

1. Krebs's calculations are cited in Mitchell HH. *Comparative Nutrition of Man and Domestic Animals*. Vol. 2. New York: Academic Press, 1964. Percent cost of digestion, p. 474; quotation, p. 541.

2. IOM. *Dietary Reference Intakes for Energy*. Washington, DC: National Academies Press, 2002:107–264.

3. Mitchell, 1964:539.

4. Livesey G. A perspective on food energy standards for nutrition labeling. *British J Nutrition* 2001;85:271–87.

5. FAO. *Food Energy—Methods of Analysis and Conversion Factors* (Food and Nutrition Paper 77). Report of a technical workshop, Rome, 3–6 December 2002, 2003:35.

6. FAO, 2003:56.

8. THE THIRD USE: PHYSICAL ACTIVITY

1. Haskell WL, et al. Physical activity and public health: Updated recommendation for adults from the American College of Sports Medicine and the American Heart Association. *Medicine and Science in Sports and Exercise* 2007;39:1423–34.

2. Atwater WO, Langworthy CF. *A Digest of Metabolism Experiments in Which the Balance of Income and Outgo Was Determined*. Washington, DC: USDA, Office of Experiment Stations, 1897. Atwater WO. *Foods: Nutritive Value and Cost*. USDA Farmers' Bull No. 23, 1894. Atwater WO. Food and diet. In: *Yearbook, United States Department of Agriculture*. Washington, DC: USDA, 1894:357–88. We estimated the calories in table 10 from the bar graph in the 1894 yearbook (table 82) and from averages given in table 1 in the 1894 Farmers' Bulletin.

3. Physiologists have their own language for reporting the results of oxygen uptake experiments. They do not report results in calories. Instead, they use the term *metabolic equivalents* (METs). METs are rates of oxygen uptake per minute corrected for body weight, sustained by a rate of oxygen consumption of 3.5 ml/kg body weight/min. At a body weight of 125 pounds, 1 MET equals 1.0 calorie per minute

(as given in table 10). But at a body weight of 155 pounds, 1 MET equals 1.2 calories, reflecting the higher energy requirement. These numbers are derived like so: 1 liter of oxygen corresponds to about 5 calories, or 0.005 calorie per ml, and 1 MET is defined as 3.5 ml of oxygen/kg/min in adults. Therefore a MET is also 0.0175 kcal/kg/min (3.5 × 0.005). For a 70 kg (155 lb) person, the calculation is 70 × 0.0175 = 1.225 METS. For a 57 kg (125 lb) person, it's 57 × 0.0175 = 0.9975 MET. See table 10 in the chapter and IOM. *Dietary Reference Intakes for Energy, Carbohydrate, Fiber, Fat, Fatty Acids, Cholesterol, Protein, and Amino Acids.* Washington, DC: National Academies Press, 2005:880–935.

4. Ainsworth BE, et al. *The Compendium of Physical Activities Tracking Guide.* Healthy Lifestyles Research Center, Arizona State University, 2011, online at https://sites.google.com/site/compendiumofphysicalactivities.

5. Black AE, et al. Human energy expenditure in affluent societies: An analysis of 574 doubly labeled water measurements. *European J Clinical Nutrition* 1995;49:72–92.

6. IOM, 2005:880–935.

7. Johannsen DL, Ravussin E. Spontaneous physical activity: Relationship between fidgeting and body weight control. *Current Opinion in Endocrinology, Diabetes, and Obesity* 2008;15:409–15. Thorburn AW, Proietto J. Biological determinants of spontaneous physical activity. *Obesity Reviews* 2000;1:87–94.

8. Roberts S, et al. Energy expenditure and intake in infants born to lean and overweight mothers. *NEJM* 1988;318:461–66. Tataranni PA, et al. Body weight gain in free-living Pima Indians: Effect of energy intake vs. expenditure. *Int'l J Obesity* 2003;27:1578–83.

9. Sourkes TL. On the energy cost of mental effort. *J History of the Neurosciences* 2006;15:31–47. The small energy cost of mental activity is discussed in Mitchell HH. *Comparative Nutrition of Man and Domestic Animals.* New York: Academic Press, 1962:71–74.

9. HOW MANY CALORIES DO YOU NEED?

1. WHO. *Energy and Protein Requirements.* Report of a joint FAO/WHO/UNU expert consultation. WHO Technical Report 724, 1985.

2. Normal ranges of weight for height are expressed as a body mass index (BMI) of 18.5 to 24.9. A BMI of 25 or above is defined as overweight, and anything over 30 is considered obese. The ratio of total energy expenditure (TEE) to the BMR is called the physical activity level (PAL). A PAL of 1.0 to 1.4 is considered sedentary, 1.4 to 1.6 is low-active, 1.6 to 1.9 is active, and 1.9 to 2.5 is very active. Doubly labeled water studies indicate that the average PAL falls mostly in the active category, except in the very young and old.

3. IOM. *Dietary Reference Intakes for Energy.* Washington, DC: National Academies Press, 2005:164–222.

4. Butte NF, Wong WW, Hopkinson JM. Energy requirements of lactating

women derived from doubly labeled water and milk energy output. *J Nutrition* 2001;131:53–58.

5. FDA. Food labeling; final rules. *FR* 1993;2066–2941. Quotation: p. 2131.

10. CALORIE CONFUSION: THE STRUGGLE TO ESTIMATE INTAKE

1. IOM. *Dietary Reference Intakes for Energy.* Washington, DC: National Academies Press, 2005:107–264. See also: Basiotis PP, Lino M, Dinkins JM. Consumption of food group servings: People's perceptions vs. reality. *Nutrition Insights* 20, October 2000, at www.cnpp.usda.gov.

2. Mertz W, ed. Beltsville one-year dietary intake study. *AJCN* 1984;6(suppl): 1323s–403s.

3. Kim WW, et al. Evaluation of long-term dietary intakes of adults consuming self-selected diets. *AJCN* 1984;40:1327–32. Kim WW, et al. Effect of making duplicate food collections on nutrient intakes calculated from diet records. *AJCN* 1984;40:1333–37.

4. Basiotis PP, et al. Number of days of food intake records required to estimate individual and group nutrient intakes with defined confidence. *J Nutrition* 1987;117:1638–41.

5. Investigators often use food frequency questionnaires to obtain dietary information from one hundred thousand individuals or more. These studies typically report calorie intakes much lower than those obtained in dietary surveys or measurement studies. For a review and critique of this method, see Lee R, Nieman D. *Nutritional Assessment,* 5th ed. New York: McGraw-Hill, 2009.

6. USDA. *What We Eat in America.* Data Tables, at www.ars.usda.gov/Services/ docs.htm?docid=13793.

7. Wright JD, Wang C-Y. Trends in intake of energy and macronutrients in adults from 1999–2000 through 2007–2008. National Center for Health Statistics Data Brief No. 49, November 2010.

8. USDA Economic Research Service. Data sets: Nutrient availability, at www .ers.usda.gov/Data/FoodConsumption/NutrientAvailIndex.htm.

9. USDA Economic Research Service. Data sets: Loss-adjusted food availability, at www.ers.usda.gov/Data/FoodConsumption/FoodGuideIndex.htm.

10. USDA. National Nutrient Database for Standard Reference, Release 23, December 2, 2010 at http://www.ars.usda.gov/Services/docs.htm?docid=8964.

11. Atwater's dissertation was "On the Proximate Composition of Several Varieties of American Maize," *Am J Science and Arts* 1869;47(November). For the early history of investigations of food composition and extensive food composition tables, see Atwater WO, Woods CD. *The Chemical Composition of American Food Materials.* USDA Office of Experiment Stations. Bull No. 28, 1896.

12. GAO. Food nutrition: Better guidance needed to improve reliability of USDA's food composition data (GAO/RCED-94-30). Washington, DC: GAO, October 1993.

11. SECRET CALORIES: ALCOHOL

1. Beer has a few vitamins provided by yeast. The health benefits of resveratrol, a chemical found in the skin of red grapes and, therefore, red wine, is the subject of much current investigation. In laboratory animals—but not yet in people—the intake of resveratrol is associated with the prevention of heart disease and cancer and with the extension of life. Agarwal B, Baur JA. Resveratrol and life extension. *Annals of the New York Academy of Sciences* 2011;1215:138–43.

2. Atwater WO, Langworthy CF. *A Digest of Metabolism Experiments in Which the Balance of Income and Outgo Was Determined*. Washington, DC: USDA Office of Experiment Stations, 1897. Atwater WO, Benedict FG. An experimental inquiry regarding the nutritive value of alcohol. *Memoirs of the National Academy of Sciences*, Vol. VIII, Sixth Memoir, 1902:231–397.

3. Levine HG. The Committee of Fifty and the origins of alcohol control. *J Drug Issues* 1983;Winter:95–116.

4. Atwater WO, Benedict FG, 1902:284.

5. Pauly PJ. The struggle for ignorance about alcohol: American physiologists, Wilbur Olin Atwater, and the Woman's Christian Temperance Union. *Bull History of Medicine* 1990;64(3):366–92. Carpenter KJ. The life and times of W. O. Atwater (1844–1907). *J Nutrition* 1994;124:1707s–14s.

6. Merrill AL, Watt BK. *Energy Value of Foods . . . Basis and Derivation*. USDA Agricultural Handbook No. 74, February 1973:18–24.

7. Livesey G. A perspective on food energy standards for nutrition labeling. *British J Nutrition* 2001;85:271–87. FAO. *Food Energy—Methods of Analysis and Conversion Factors* (Food and Nutrition Paper 77). Report of a technical workshop, 3–6 December 2002, Rome, 2003:56.

8. USDA. USDA National Nutrient Database for Standard Reference, Release 23, December 2, 2010, at http://www.ars.usda.gov/Services/docs.htm?docid=8964.

9. The Treasury Department's Bureau of Alcohol, Tobacco and Firearms (ATF) used to regulate alcohol. This changed in 2003 when the Homeland Security Act transferred the law enforcement functions of the ATF to the Department of Justice under a newly named Bureau of Alcohol, Tobacco, Firearms and Explosives. The tax and trade functions remained in the Department of the Treasury. Information about the TTB is at www.ttb.gov. Its regulations appear at www.ttb.gov/other/regulations.shtml.

10. When alcohol and water are mixed together, alcohol molecules fall into the spaces between water molecules. To visualize how this works, think of what would happen if you combined equal volumes of sand and rocks. Similarly, adding an ounce of alcohol to an ounce of water gives you a volume of less than two ounces.

11. Guo R, Ren J. Alcohol and acetaldehyde in public health: From marvel to menace. *Int'l J Environmental Research in Public Health* 2010;7:1285–301.

12. Lieber CS. Perspectives: Do alcohol calories count? *AJCN* 1991;54:976–82.

13. Robin A, LaVallee RA, Yi H-y. Surveillance Report No. 90. Apparent per

capita alcohol consumption, national, state, and regional trends, 1977–2008. Table 1: Apparent per capita ethanol consumption, United States, 1850–2008, National Institute on Alcohol Abuse and Alcoholism, August 2010 at http://pubs.niaaa.nih .gov/publications/Surveillance90/tab1_08.htm. WHO. *Global Status Report on Alcohol and Health*, 2011, at www.who.int/substance_abuse/publications/global_alcohol _report/en/index.html.

12. CALORIE REGULATION: THE BODY'S COMPLEX WEIGHT MANAGEMENT SYSTEM

1. See, for example, Berthoud H-R, Morrison C. The brain, appetite, and obesity. *Annual Review of Psychology* 2008;59:55–92.

2. Suzuki K, et al. The role of gut hormones and the hypothalamus in appetite regulation. *Endocrine J* 2010;57:359–72.

3. Seeley RJ, Sandoval DA. Weight loss through smoking. *Nature* 2011;475:176–77. Mineur YS, et al. Nicotine decreases food intake through activation of POMC neurons. *Science* 2011;332:1330–32.

4. Wisser A-S, et al. Interactions of gastrointestinal peptides: Ghrelin and its anorexigenic antagonists. *Int'l J Peptides* 2010:ID 817457, available at www.hindawi .com/journals/ijpep/2010/817457.html.

5. Zorrilla EP, et al. Vaccination against weight gain. *Proceedings of the National Academy of Sciences U.S.A.* 2006;103(35):13226–31. Vizcarra JA, et al. Active immunization against ghrelin decreases weight gain and alters plasma concentrations of growth hormone in growing pigs. *Domestic Animal Endocrinology* 2007;33(2):176–89.

6. Friedman JM, Halaas JL. Leptin and the regulation of body weight in mammals. *Nature* 1998;395:763–70.

7. Heymsfeld SB, et al. Recombinant leptin for weight loss in obese and lean adults: A randomized, controlled, dose-escalation trial. *JAMA* 1999;282:1568–75. Havel PJ. Peripheral signals conveying metabolic information to the brain: Short-term and long-term regulation of food intake and energy homeostasis. *Experimental Biology and Medicine* 2001;226:963–77.

8. Friedman J. Leptin at 14 y of age: An ongoing story. *AJCN* 2009;89(suppl): 973s–79s.

9. Levitsky DA. The non-regulation of food intake in humans: Hope for reversing the epidemic of obesity. *Physiology and Behavior* 2005;86:623–32. Bennett W, Gurin J. *The Dieter's Dilemma: Eating Less and Weighing More*. New York: Basic Books, 1982. Blackburn G, Corliss J. *Break Through Your Set Point: How to Finally Lose the Weight You Want and Keep It Off*. New York: William Morrow, 2008.

10. Levitsky DA. Putting behavior back into feeding behavior: A tribute to George Collier. *Appetite* 2002;38:143–48.

11. Comuzzie AG. The emerging pattern of the genetic contribution to human obesity. *Best Practice and Res: Clinical Endocrinology and Metabolism* 2002;16:611–21.

Farooqi S, O'Rahilly S. Genetics of obesity in humans. *Endocrine Reviews* 2006;27:710–18.

12. Prentice AM, Henning BJ, Fulford AJ. Evolutionary origins of the obesity epidemic: Natural selection of thrifty genes or genetic drift following predation release? *Int'l J Obesity* 2008;32:1607–10.

13. National Diabetes Information Clearinghouse. The Pima Indians: Pathfinders for health, May 2002, at http://diabetes.niddk.nih.gov/dm/pubs/pima/index.htm.

14. Speakman JR. Thrifty genes for obesity, an attractive but flawed idea, and an alternative perspective: The "drifty gene" hypothesis. *Int'l J Obesity* 2008;32: 1601–07.

15. Leibel RL. Energy in, energy out, and the effects of obesity-related genes. *NEJM* 2008;359:2603–04.

16. Sumithran P, et al. Long-term persistence of hormonal adaptations to weight loss. *NEJM* 2011;365:1597–1604. Friedman J, 2009: 977s.

17. Kessler DA. *The End of Overeating*. Emmaus, PA: Rodale Press, 2009. Schwartz MW, et al. Is the energy homeostasis system inherently biased toward weight gain? *Diabetes* 2003;52:232–38. De Castro JM. The control of food intake of free-living humans: Putting the pieces back together. *Physiology and Behavior* 2010;100:446–53.

13. STARVATION AND ITS EFFECTS ON THE BODY

1. Winick M, ed. *Hunger Disease: Studies by Jewish Physicians in the Warsaw Ghetto*. New York: John Wiley and Sons, 1979.

2. Kerndt PR, et al. Fasting: The history, pathophysiology and complications. *Western J Medicine* 1982;137:379–99.

3. The purpose of the strike was to obtain the right to be considered political—rather than common—prisoners. Sands was elected to the Irish Parliament while undergoing his fatal fast, and 90,000 people attended his funeral. See: Beresford D. *Ten Men Dead: The Story of the 1981 Irish Hunger Strike*. New York: Atlantic Monthly Press, 1987. See also: Collins T. *The Irish Hunger Strike*. Dublin: White Island Book Co., 1986.

4. Keys A, Brozek J, Henschel A. *The Biology of Human Starvation*. Minneapolis: U Minnesota Press, 1950. Keys was already known for studies of high-altitude physiology and the development of K rations during World War II. Later he led the Seven Countries Study comparing the health effects of dietary patterns, such as Mediterranean. He died at the age of 100 in 2004.

5. Men starve in Minnesota: Conscientious objectors volunteer for strict hunger tests to study Europe's food problem. *Life*, July 30, 1945:43–46.

6. Tucker T. *The Great Starvation Experiment*. Minneapolis: U Minnesota Press, 2006. Tucker interviewed the surviving participants in the Minnesota study and reports their reflections on how it felt at the time and what it meant to them in retrospect.

7. Kreitzman SN, Coxon AY, Szaz KF. Glycogen storage: Illusions of easy weight loss, excessive weight regain, and distortions in estimates of body composition. *AJCN* 1992;56:292s–93s.

14. INDIVIDUALS, COMMUNITIES, NATIONS: CALORIES AND GLOBAL HUNGER

1. FAO. *The State of Food Insecurity in the World, 2010.* Rome, FAO, October 2010, available at www.fao.org.

2. FAO hunger statistics are at www.fao.org/hunger/en/. See also: Hunger: Frequently asked questions, at www.fao.org/hunger/faqs-on-hunger/en/.

3. USDA economists perform similar estimates but set the minimal intake level 300 calories higher—at 2,100 calories per day. By USDA calculations, 882 million people were expected to lack adequate food in 2010. The USDA estimate is lower than that of the FAO despite using a higher calorie threshold, perhaps because the USDA includes expected food aid in the per capita calorie availability. See: Shapouri S, et al. *Food Security Assessment, 2010–20.* USDA Outlook Report GFA-21, July 2010. See also: WHO. *Energy and Protein Requirements.* Report of a joint FAO/WHO/UNU expert consultation. WHO Technical Report 724, 1985.

4. The FAOSTAT Food Balance Sheets may be accessed at http://faostat.fao.org/site/354/default.aspx. The figures from 2007 were the most recent available in 2011.

5. Dewey KG, Brown KH. Update on technical issues concerning complementary feeding of young children in developing countries . . . *Food and Nutrition Bull* 2003;24:5–28. Dror DK, Allen LH. The importance of milk and other animal-source foods for children in low-income countries. *Food and Nutrition Bull* 2011;32:227–43.

6. Williams CD. Kwashiorkor: A nutritional disease of children associated with a maize diet. *Lancet* 1935;226:1151–52.

7. McLaren DS. The great protein fiasco. *Lancet* 1974;304:93–96.

8. UNICEF. Childinfo: Monitoring the situation of children and women: Statistics by area / Child nutrition: Undernutrition: Current status, at www.childinfo.org/undernutrition_status.html.

9. Black RF, et al. Maternal and child undernutrition: Global and regional exposures and health consequences. *Lancet* 2008;371:243–60. Caulfield LE, et al. Undernutrition as an underlying cause of child deaths associated with diarrhea, pneumonia, malaria and measles. *AJCN* 2004;80:193–98.

10. Csete J, Nestle M. Global nutrition: Complex aetiology demands social as well as nutrient-based solutions. In: Parker R, Sommer M, eds. *Routledge Handbook of Global Public Health.* New York: Routledge, 2011:303–13.

11. Millennium Development Goal Monitor. Eradicate extreme poverty and hunger (MDG monitor tool), 2009, at www.mdgmonitor.org/goal1.cfm.

12. UNICEF. *Strategy for Improved Nutrition of Children and Women in Developing Countries.* New York: UNICEF, 1990.

13. Bhutta ZA, et al. What works? Interventions for maternal and child under-

nutrition and survival. *Lancet* 2008;371:417–40. WHO. Nutrition: Nutrition health topics: Complementary feeding, at www.who.int/nutrition/topics/complementary _feeding/en/. Labbok MH, Clark D, Goldman AS. Breastfeeding: Maintaining an irreplaceable immunological resource. *Nature Reviews Immunology* 2004;4:565–72. Martorell R, et al. The nutrition intervention improved adult human capital and economic productivity. *J Nutrition* 2010;140:411–14.

14. WHO, World Food Programme, United Nations System Standing Committee on Nutrition, United Nations Children's Fund. Community-based management of severe acute malnutrition, 2007, available at www.who.int/child_adolescent _health/documents/a91065/en/.

15. Rice A. The peanut solution. *NYT Magazine*, September 2, 2010.

16. Von Grebmer K, et al. *2010 Global Hunger Index: The Challenge of Hunger: Focus on the Crisis of Child Undernutrition*. Washington, DC: International Food Policy Research Institute, October 2010.

17. Nestle M. Hunger in America: A matter of policy. *Social Res* 1999;66(1):257–82.

18. USDA Economic Research Service. Data sets: Nutrient availability, February 1, 2010, at www.ers.usda.gov/Data/FoodConsumption/NutrientAvailIndex.htm.

19. USDA Economic Research Service. Briefing rooms: Food security in the United States, updated November 15, 2010, at www.ers.usda.gov/Briefing/Food Security/. Coleman-Jenson A, et al. *Household Food Security in the United States, 2010.* USDA Economic Research Service, Economic Research Report No. 125, November 2010, available at www.ers.usda.gov/publications/err125/. USDA Food and Nutrition Service. Nutrition assistance programs, at www.fns.usda.gov/fns/.

15. COULD RESTRICTING CALORIES PROLONG HUMAN LIFE?

1. McCay C, Cowell M, Maynard LA. The effect of retarded growth upon length of life and upon ultimate size. *J Nutrition* 1935;10:63–79. McCay C, et al. Retarded growth, life span, ultimate body size and age changes in the albino rat after feeding diets restricted in calories. *J Nutrition* 1939;18:1–13.

2. Masoro EJ. Caloric restriction and aging: An update. *Experimental Gerontology* 2000;35:299–303. Morley JE, Chahla E, Alkaade S. Antiaging, longevity, and calorie restriction. *Current Opinion in Clinical Nutrition and Metabolic Care* 2010;13:40–45. Lawler DF. Influence of lifetime food restriction on causes, time, and predictors of death in dogs. *J Am Veterinary Medical Association* 2005;226:225–31.

3. Colman RJ, et al. Caloric restriction delays disease onset and mortality in rhesus monkeys. *Science* 2009;325:201–4.

4. Bodkin NL, et al. Mortality and morbidity in laboratory-maintained rhesus monkeys and effects of long-term dietary restriction. *J Gerontology: Biological Sciences* 2003;58:212–19. Ingram DK, et al. The potential for dietary restriction to increase longevity in humans: Extrapolation from monkey studies. *Biogerontology* 2006;7:143–48.

5. Wilcox DC, et al. Caloric restriction and human longevity: What can we learn

from the Okinawans? *Biogerontology* 2006;7:173–77. The average body mass index of the Okinawans was 21, at the low end of the range considered optimal in the United States (see chapter 16).

6. Redman LM, et al. Effect of calorie restriction with and without exercise on body composition and fat distribution. *J Clinical Endocrinology and Metabolism* 2007;92:865–72.

7. Heilbronn LK, et al. Effect of 6-month calorie restriction on biomarkers of longevity, metabolic adaptation, and oxidative stress in overweight individuals—a randomized controlled trial. *JAMA* 2006;295:1539–48.

8. National Institute on Aging. Scientists weigh mechanisms, effects of calorie restriction. *Spotlight on Aging Research,* E-zine, March 2008, at www.nia.nih.gov/NewsAndEvents/SOAR/viii/DiscoveryInnovation/calorie.htm. Rochon J, et al. CALERIE Study Group. Design and conduct of the CALERIE study: Comprehensive assessment of the long-term effects of reducing intake of energy. *J Gerontology: Biological Sciences* 2011;66(1):97–108.

9. Gertner J. The calorie-restriction experiment. *NYT Magazine,* October 7, 2009.

10. Keys A, Brozek J, Henschel A. *The Biology of Human Starvation.* Minneapolis: U Minnesota Press, 1950.

11. Calorie Restriction Society, www.crsociety.org. Quote: History of the CR Society, at www.crsociety.org/History. See Weindruch R, et al. The retardation of aging in mice by dietary restriction: Longevity, cancer, immunity and lifetime energy intake. *J Nutrition* 1986;116:641–54.

12. Fontana L, et al. Long-term calorie restriction is highly effective in reducing the risk for atherosclerosis in humans. *Proceedings of the National Academy of Sciences U.S.A.* 2004;101:6659–63.

13. Allday E. UCSF study takes closer look at calorie restrictors. *San Francisco Chronicle,* April 28, 2011.

14. Huang C, et al. Early life exposure to the 1959–61 Chinese famine has long-term health consequences. *J Nutrition* 2010;140:1874–78. Li Y, et al. Exposure to the Chinese famine in early life and the risk of hyperglycemia and type 2 diabetes in adulthood. *Diabetes* 2010;59(10):2400–2406. Numerous studies report higher levels of age-related diseases among adults whose mothers experienced semistarvation during pregnancy, but their relevance to calorie restriction in adults is uncertain. See, for example: Barker DJ, et al. The early origins of chronic heart failure: Impaired placental growth and initiation of insulin resistance in childhood. *European J Heart Failure* 2010;12(8):819–25.

15. Flegal KM, et al. Cause-specific excess deaths associated with underweight, overweight, and obesity. *JAMA* 2007;298:2028–37.

16. Le Bourg E, Rattan SIS. Can calorie restriction increase longevity in all species, particularly in human beings? *Biogerontology* 2006;7:123–25. Everitt AV, LeCouteur DG. Life extension by calorie restriction in humans. *Annals of the New York Academy of Sciences* 2007;1114:428–33. This review concludes that overweight

(defined here as BMI 25–30) shortens life by 3 years, obesity (BMI >30) by 7 years, and very extreme obesity (BMI >45) by 13 years. Adams KF, et al. Overweight, obesity, and mortality in a large prospective cohort of persons 50 to 71 years old. *NEJM* 2006;355:763–68.

17. Minor RK, et al. Dietary interventions to extend life span and health span based on calorie restriction. *J Gerontology: Biological Sciences* 2010;65:695–703. Chachay VS, et al. Resveratrol—pills to replace a healthy diet? *British J Clinical Pharmacology* 2011;72:27–38.

16. AN INTRODUCTION TO OBESITY

1. CDC. Adult BMI calculator: English, at www.cdc.gov/healthyweight/assessing/bmi/adult_bmi/english_bmi_calculator/bmi_calculator.html. The BMI calculator for children is at http://apps.nccd.cdc.gov/dnpabmi.

2. Body fat content can be measured in population surveys via skinfold thickness (with calipers), but the method is not accurate enough for research purposes. Other methods—underwater weighing, bioelectrical impedance, dual-energy x-ray absorption, and isotope dilution—are more accurate but require skill to conduct and interpret and are expensive, difficult to standardize, and inconvenient for large-scale surveys of populations.

3. Prospective Studies Collaboration. Body-mass index and cause-specific mortality in 900,000 adults: Collaborative analyses of 57 prospective studies. *Lancet* 2009;373:1083–96. Mortality risks also increase at BMIs below the normal range, resulting in a J-shaped curve, meaning that mortality increases at body weights below as well as above the range considered normal.

4. CDC. Overweight and obesity: Health consequences, at www.cdc.gov/obesity/causes/health.html.

5. Grundy SM, et al. Definition of metabolic syndrome. *Circulation* 2004; 109:433–38. Finkelstein EA, et al. Annual medical spending attributable to obesity: Payer- and service-specific estimates. *Health Affairs* 2009;28:w822–w831. Cawley J, Meyerhoefer C. The medical care costs of obesity: An instrumental variables approach. National Bureau of Economic Research Working Paper No. 16467, 2010, available at www.nber.org/papers/w16467.

6. Grundy SM, et al. Clinical management of metabolic syndrome. *Circulation* 2004;109:551–56. USDA, HHS. *Dietary Guidelines for Americans, 2010.* Washington, DC: U.S. Dept. of Agriculture.

7. Flegal KM, et al. Overweight and obesity in the United States: Prevalence and trends, 1960–1994. *JAMA* 1994;272:205–11. Flegal KM, et al. Prevalence and trends in obesity among US adults, 1999–2008. *JAMA* 2010;303:235–41. CDC. NCHS Health E-Stat: Prevalence of overweight, obesity and extreme obesity among adults: United States, trends 1960–62 through 2005–2006, at www.cdc.gov/nchs/data/hestat/overweight/overweight_adult.htm.

8. Ogden CL, et al. Mean body weight height and body mass index, United

States, 1960–2002. *Advance Data from Vital and Health Statistics*, No. 347, October 27, 2004.

9. Hill AL, et al. Infectious disease modeling of social contagion in networks. *PLoS Computational Biology* 2010;6(11):e1000968. doi:10.1371/journal.pcbi.1000968. Wang YC, et al. Health and economic burden of the projected obesity trends in the USA and the UK. *Lancet* 2011;378:815–25.

10. CDC. Overweight and obesity: Basics about childhood obesity: How is childhood overweight and obesity measured? at www.cdc.gov/obesity/childhood/basics.html. McDowell MA, et al. Anthropometric data for children and adults: United States, 2003–2006. *National Health Statistics Reports*, No. 10, October 22, 2008.

11. Ogden C, Carroll M. NCHS Health E-Stat: Prevalence of obesity among children and adolescents: United States, trends 1963–1965 through 2007–2008, updated June 2010, at www.cdc.gov/nchs/data/hestat/obesity_child_07_08/obesity_child_07_08.htm.

12. Finucane MM, et al. National, regional, and global trends in body-mass index since 1980: Systematic analysis of health examination surveys and epidemiological studies with 960 country years and 9.1 million participants. *Lancet* 2011;377:557–67. WHO. Health topics: Obesity, at www.who.int/topics/obesity/en/.

17. CALORIES AND WEIGHT GAIN: ANOTHER COMPLEX RELATIONSHIP

1. See, for example: *Dimensions* magazine. The world's heaviest people, at www.dimensionsmagazine.com/dimtext/kjn/people/heaviest.htm.

2. Stewart WK, Fleming LA. Features of a successful therapeutic fast of 382 days' duration. *Postgraduate Medical J* 1973;49:203–9.

3. Arner P, Spalding KL. Fat cell turnover in humans. *Biochemical and Biophysical Research Communications* 2010;396:101–04. Heymsfield S, Baumgartner RN. Body composition and anthropometry. In: Shils M, et al., eds. *Modern Nutrition in Health and Disease*, 10th ed. Baltimore, MD: Lippincott, Williams and Wilkins, 2006:751–70.

4. Jebb SA, et al. Changes in macronutrient balance during over- and under-feeding assessed by 12-d continuous whole-body calorimetry. *AJCN* 1996;64:259–66. New York City Department of Health and Mental Hygiene. Press release: Health Department's new TV spot shows how a day's worth of sugary drinks adds up to a whopping 93 sugar packets, January 31, 2011, at http://home2.nyc.gov/html/doh/html/pr2011/pr001–11.shtml.

5. Sims EA, et al. Experimental obesity in man. *Transactions of the Association of Am Physicians* 1968;81:153–70.

6. Hill JO, et al. Obesity and the environment: Where do we go from here? *Science* 2003:299:853–55.

7. USDA, National Institute of Food and Agriculture. America on the Move

and the Cooperative Extension Service: Partners for healthy living, available at www .nifa.usda.gov/nea/food/pdfs/AOM_NIFA_trifold.pdf. America on the Move is described at www.csrees.usda.gov/nea/food/part/health_part_aom.html.

8. Butte NF, Ellis KJ. Comment on "Obesity and the environment: Where do we go from here?" *Science* 2003;301:598.

9. IOM. *Dietary Reference Intakes for Energy*. Washington, DC: National Academies Press, 2005.

10. Hall KD, Jordan PN. Modeling weight-loss maintenance to help prevent body weight regain. *AJCN* 2008;88:1495–503. Swinburn BA, et al. Estimating the changes in energy flux that characterize the rise in obesity prevalence. *AJCN* 2009;89:1723–28.

11. Swinburn B, Sacks G, Ravussin E. Increased food energy supply is more than sufficient to explain the US epidemic of obesity. *AJCN* 2009;90:1453–56. The Body Weight Simulator accompanies a series of articles in *Lancet* on obesity policy, August 26, 2011, online at www.thelancet.com/series/obesity.

12. Katan MB, Ludwig DS. Extra calories cause weight gain—but how much? *JAMA* 2010;303:65–66. Wang YC, et al. Estimating the energy gap among US children: A counterfactual approach. *Pediatrics* 2006;118:e1721–33.

18. DO EXCESS CALORIES MAKE SOME PEOPLE GAIN WEIGHT FASTER THAN OTHERS?

1. Levine JA, Eberhardt NL, Jensen MD. Role of nonexercise activity thermogenesis in resistance to fat gain in humans. *Science* 1999;283:212–14. See also: commentary by Ravussin E, Danforth E, Jr. Beyond sloth—physical activity and weight gain. *Science* 1999;283:184–85. Bouchard C, et al. The response to overfeeding in identical twins. *NEJM* 1990;322:1477–82.

2. Joosen A, Westerterp KR. Energy expenditure during overfeeding. *Nutrition and Metabolism* 2006;3:25, available at www.nutritionandmetabolism.com/content/3/1/25.

3. Rothwell NJ, Stock MJ. A role for brown adipose tissue in diet-induced thermogenesis. *Nature* 1979;281:31–35.

4. Celi FS. Brown adipose tissue—when it pays to be inefficient. *NEJM* 2009;360:1553–57.

5. Levine JA, Eberhardt NL, Jensen MD, 1999.

6. Ravussin E, et al. Determinants of 24-hour energy expenditure in man. *J Clinical Investigation* 1986;78:1569–78. The NIH calorimeter was an 88-square-foot space complete with bed, sink, toilet, desk, and sitting area.

7. Garland G, et al. The biological control of voluntary exercise, spontaneous physical activity and daily energy expenditure in relation to obesity: Human and rodent perspectives. *J Experimental Biology* 2011;214:208–29.

8. Johannsen DL, Ravussin E. Spontaneous physical activity: Relationship

between fidgeting and body weight control. *Current Opinion in Endocrinology, Diabetes, and Obesity* 2008;15:409–15. Benden ME, et al. The impact of stand-biased desks in classrooms on calorie expenditure in children. *Am J Public Health* 2011;101:1433–36.

9. Rao J. It's the year of the value diet, June 18, 2010, at www.cnbc.com/id/37492840/It_s_The_Year_of_The_Value_Diet. The diet industries figure comes from a report from MarketData Enterprises at MarketResearch.com.

10. Bish CL, et al. Diet and physical activity behaviors among Americans trying to lose weight: 2000 Behavioral Risk Factor Surveillance System. *Obesity Res* 2005;13:596–607.

11. Deutsch RM. *The New Nuts among the Berries.* Palo Alto, CA: Bull, 1977. Yager S. *The Hundred Year Diet: America's Voracious Appetite for Losing Weight.* Emmaus, PA: Rodale, 2010.

12. Peters LH. *Diet and Health with Key to the Calories.* Chicago: Reilly and Lee, 1918. Peters lived from 1873 to 1930. Mary Baker Eddy (1821–1910), the founder of Christian Science, first published *Science and Health* in 1875; it remains in print.

13. Peters LH, 1918:84.

14. Kraschnewski JL, et al. Long-term weight loss maintenance in the United States. *Int'l J Obesity* 2010;34:1644–54. Anderson JW, et al. Long-term weight-loss maintenance: A meta-analysis of US studies. *AJCN* 2001;74:579–84.

15. Wing RR, Hill JO. Successful weight maintenance. *Annual Review of Nutrition* 2001;21:323–41. The National Weight Control Registry is at www.nwcr.ws.

16. Kreitzman SN, Coxon AY, Szaz KF. Glycogen storage: Illusions of easy weight loss, excessive weight regain, and distortions in estimates of body composition. *AJCN* 1992;56:292s–93s.

19. ARE ALL CALORIES CREATED EQUAL?

1. Kinsell LW, et al. Calories do count. *Metabolism: Clinical and Experimental* 1964;13:195–204.

2. Park M. Twinkie diet helps nutrition professor lose 27 pounds, November 8, 2010, at www.cnn.com/2010/HEALTH/11/08/twinkie.diet.professor/index.html. Katz D. "Twinkie Diet": A physician's take on what really happens, November 13, 2010, at www.huffingtonpost.com/david-katz-md/chewing-on-the-twinkie-di_b_782678.html.

3. Stillman IM. *The Doctor's Quick Weight Loss Diet.* Englewood Cliffs, NJ: Prentice Hall, 1967. Atkins RC. *Dr. Atkins' Diet Revolution.* New York: Bantam, 1981.

4. Bravata DM, et al. Efficacy and safety of low-carbohydrate diets: A systemic review. *JAMA* 2003;289:1837–50. Astrup A, et al. Atkins and other low-carbohydrate diets: Hoax or an effective tool for weight loss? *Lancet* 2004;364:897–99. But see: Sjögren P, et al. Mediterranean and carbohydrate-restricted diets and mortality among elderly men: A cohort study in Sweden. *AJCN* 2010;92:967–74. In this

study of elderly Swedish men, the men on the carbohydrate-restricted diet displayed *increased* mortality compared to men consuming a Mediterranean-type diet.

5. Crowe TC. Safety of low-carbohydrate diets. *Obesity Reviews* 2005;6:235–45. Wylie-Rosett J, Davis NJ. Low-carbohydrate diets: An update on current research. *Current Diabetes Reports* 2009;9:396–404.

6. Jenkins DJA, et al. Glycemic index of foods: A physiological basis for carbohydrate exchange. *AJCN* 1981;34:362–66.

7. Ludwig DS. The glycemic index—physiological mechanisms relating to obesity, diabetes, and cardiovascular disease. *JAMA* 2002;287:2414–23.

8. Taubes G. *Good Calories, Bad Calories.* New York: Random House, 2008:xxiii. See also: Taubes G. *Why We Get Fat.* New York: Knopf, 2010. And see Wells JCK, Siervo M. Obesity and energy balance: Is the tail wagging the dog? *European J Clinical Nutrition* 2011;1–17 doi:10:1038/ejcn.2011.132.

9. IOM. *Dietary Reference Intakes for Energy.* Washington, DC: National Academies Press, 2005.

10. Bray GA. Viewpoint: *Good Calories, Bad Calories* by Gary Taubes. New York: AA Knopf. *Obesity Reviews* 2008;9:251–63. Freedhoff Y. Book review: Gary Taubes' *Why We Get Fat. Weighty Matters* (blog), January 10, 2011, at www.weighty matters.ca/2011/01/book-review-gary-taubes-why-we-get-fat.html.

11. USDA. Added sugar and sweeteners, February 1, 2010, available at Food availability: Spreadsheets, at www.ers.usda.gov/Data/FoodConsumption/Food AvailSpreadsheets.htm. Whether the difference between the 55 percent fructose in HFCS and the 50 percent fructose in sucrose is biologically meaningful is uncertain. But one point is clear: people would be better off eating a lot less of either one.

12. Duffey KJ, Popkin BM. Shifts in patterns and consumptions of beverages between 1965 and 2002. *Obesity* 2007;15:2739–47. Bray GA. Soft drink consumption and obesity: It is all about fructose. *Current Opinion in Lipidology* 2010;21:51–57. See also: Vos MB, et al. Dietary fructose consumption among US children and adults: The Third National Health and Nutrition Examination Survey. *Medscape J Medicine* 2008;10:160, published online at www.ncbi.nlm.nih.gov/pmc/articles/PMC 2525476/?tool=pmcentrez.

13. Bray GA, Nielsen SJ, Popkin BM. Consumption of high-fructose corn syrup in beverages may play a role in the epidemic of obesity. *AJCN* 2004;79:537–43.

14. Lim JS, et al. The role of fructose in the pathogenesis of NAFLD and the metabolic syndrome. *Nature Reviews Gastroenterology and Hepatology* 2010;7:251–64.

15. Mattes RD. Dietary compensation by humans for supplemental energy provided as ethanol or carbohydrate in fluids. *Physiology and Behavior* 1996;59:179–87. Malik VS, Schulze MB, Hu FB. Intake of sugar-sweetened beverages and weight gain: A systematic review. *AJCN* 2006;84:274–88. Malik VS, et al. Sugar-sweetened beverages and risk of metabolic syndrome and type 2 diabetes. *Diabetes Care* 2010; 33:2477–83.

20. DO SOME KINDS OF DIETS WORK BETTER THAN OTHERS?

1. Atkins RC. *Dr. Atkins' New Diet Revolution*. New York: Avon Books, 2002 (this is the version current at the time of this writing). Agatston A. *The South Beach Diet*. Emmaus, PA: Rodale, 2003. Ornish D. *Eat More, Weigh Less: Dr. Dean Ornish's Life Choice Program for Losing Weight Safely while Eating Abundantly*. New York: HarperTorch, 2001.

2. Winkler JT. The fundamental flaw in obesity research. *Obesity Reviews* 2005; 6:199–202.

3. Bray GA, Popkin BM. Dietary fat intake does affect obesity! *AJCN* 1998; 68:1157–73.

4. Willett WC. Dietary fat and obesity: An unconvincing relation. *AJCN* 1998;68:1149–50. Forouhi NG, et al. Dietary fat intake and subsequent weight change in adults: Results from the European Prospective Investigation into Cancer and Nutrition cohorts. *AJCN* 2009;90:1632–41.

5. Due A, et al. Comparison of 3 ad libitum diets for weight-loss maintenance, risk of cardiovascular disease, and diabetes: A 6-mo randomized, controlled trial. *AJCN* 2008;88:1232–41.

6. Carty CL, et al. Low-fat dietary pattern and change in body-composition traits in the Women's Health Initiative Dietary Modification Trial. *AJCN* 2011;93:516–24. For a comment on the importance of adherence, see: Bray GA. Is dietary fat important? *AJCN* 2011;93:481–82.

7. Mikkelsen PB, Toubro S, Astrup A. Effect of fat-reduced diets on 24-h energy expenditure: Comparisons between animal protein, vegetable protein, and carbohydrate. *AJCN* 2000;72:1135–41. Eisenstein J, et al. High-protein weight-loss diets: Are they safe and do they work? A review of the experimental and epidemiologic data. *Nutrition Reviews* 2002;60:189–200.

8. Halton TL, Hu FB. The effects of high protein diets on thermogenesis, satiety and weight loss: A critical review. *J Am College of Nutrition* 2004;23:373–85.

9. Freedman MK, King J, Kennedy E. Popular diets: A scientific review. *Obesity* 2001;9(suppl 1):1s–40s. Weight Watchers' PointsPlus lets dieters eat anything they like as long as they do not exceed a daily point allotment. The system assigns zero points to fruits and vegetables. Weight Watchers maintains a network of weight-loss centers and sells food products and online subscriptions. See www.weightwatchers.com/plan/eat/index.aspx.

10. Gardner CD, et al. Comparison of the Atkins, Zone, Ornish, and LEARN diets for change in weight and related risk factors among overweight premenopausal women. *JAMA* 2007;297:969–77.

11. Sacks FM, et al. Comparison of weight-loss diets with different compositions of fat, protein, and carbohydrates. *NEJM* 2009;360:859–73.

12. Larsen TM, et al. Diets with high or low protein content and glycemic index for weight-loss maintenance. *NEJM* 2010;363:2102–13. See also: Ludwig D, Ebbeling C. Weight-loss maintenance—mind over matter? *NEJM* 2010;363:2159–61.

13. Foster GD, et al. Weight and metabolic outcomes after 2 years on a low-carbohydrate versus low-fat diet. *Annals of Internal Medicine* 2010;153:147–57.

14. Fung T, et al. Low-carbohydrate diets and all-cause and cause-specific mortality—two cohort studies. *Annals of Internal Medicine* 2010;153:289–98.

15. USDA and HHS. *Report of the Dietary Guidelines Advisory Committee on the Dietary Guidelines for Americans, 2010*. Washington, DC: USDA, 2010:98.

16. Friedman J. A war on obesity, not the obese. *Science* 2003;299:856–58.

17. Kessler DA. *The End of Overeating*. Emmaus, PA: Rodale, 2009.

21. TODAY'S "EAT MORE" ENVIRONMENT: THE ROLE OF THE FOOD INDUSTRY

1. Blair SN, Leermaker EA. Exercise and weight management. In: Wadden TA, Stunkard AJ, eds. *Handbook of Obesity Treatment*. New York: Guilford Press, 2004:283–300. Church TS, et al. Trends over 5 decades in U.S. occupation-related physical activity and their associations with obesity. *PLoS One* 2011;6(5):e19657.

2. Westerterp KR, Speakman JR. Physical activity energy expenditure has not declined since the 1980s and matches energy expenditures of wild animals. *Int'l J Obesity* 2008;32:1256–63. CDC. Physical activity trends—United States, 1990–1998. *Morbidity and Mortality Weekly Report* 2001;50:166–69. CDC. Physical activity statistics, updated February 2, 2010, at www.cdc.gov/nccdphp/dnpa/physical/stats/.

3. CDC. Prevalence of regular physical activity among adults—United States, 2001 and 2005. *Morbidity and Mortality Weekly Report* 2007;56:1209–12. Adams J. Trends in physical activity and inactivity amongst US 14–18 year olds by gender, school grade and race, 1993–2003: Evidence from the youth risk behavior survey. *BMC Public Health* 2006;6:57, online at www.biomedcentral.com/1471-2458/6/57. Kimm SYS, et al. Decline in physical activity in black girls and white girls during adolescence. *NEJM* 2002;347:709–15. Dollman J, Norton K, Norton L. Evidence for secular trends in children's physical activity behavior. *British J Sports Medicine* 2005;39:892–97.

4. Tataranni PA, et al. Body weight gain in free-living Pima Indians: Effect of energy intake vs. expenditure. *Int'l J Obesity* 2003;27:1578–83.

5. CDC. Trends in intake of energy and macronutrients—United States, 1971–2000. *Morbidity and Mortality Weekly Report* 2004;53:80–82.

6. USDA. Data tables from *What We Eat in America*, NHANES 2007–2008, revised August 2010, available at www.ars.usda.gov/Services/docs.htm?docid=18349. Kant AK, Graubard BI. Secular trends in patterns of self-reported food consumption of American adults: NHANES 1971–1975 to NHANES 1999–2002. *AJCN* 2006;84:1215–23.

7. Swinburn BA, Sacks G, Ravussin E. Increased food energy supply is more than sufficient to explain the US epidemic of obesity. *AJCN* 2009;90:1453–56.

8. Percentages are calculated using Atwater Values from figures in the USDA Food Availability (Per Capita) Data System, at www.ers.usda.gov/data/foodconsumption.

These data show no change in the availability of sugars as a percent of calories from 1980 to 2000. The data sets do not distinguish whole from refined grains, but daily fiber availability increased by 5 grams per day during that period, perhaps indicating some increase in the availability of whole grains.

9. USDA, HHS. *Dietary Guidelines for Americans*, 2010, at www.dietaryguide lines.gov. The NHANES data are analyzed in National Cancer Institute. Food sources of energy among U.S. population, 2005–06. National Cancer Institute, May 21, 2010, at http://riskfactor.cancer.gov/diet/foodsources.

10. Ogden CL, et al. Consumption of sugar drinks in the United States, 2005–2008. NCHS Data Brief No. 71, August 2011, at www.cdc.gov/nchs/data/databriefs/db71.htm.

11. Rupert P, Stepanczuk C. Economic trends: Women in the workforce. Federal Reserve Bank of Cleveland website, March 15, 2007, at www.clevelandfed.org/research/trends/2007/0407/03ecoact_031407.cfm.

12. Breimyer HF. *Over-fulfilled Expectations: A Life in Rural America*. Ames: Iowa State U Press, 1991. USDA, Economic Research Service. Data sets: Loss-adjusted food availability: Spreadsheets, updated March 17, 2010, at www.ers.usda.gov/data/foodconsumption/FoodGuideSpreadsheets.htm.

13. Morris B. The new rules. *Fortune*, July 24, 2006. Welch's speech was titled "Growing Fast in a Slow-Growth Economy." The shareholder value movement is usually traced to the work of Alfred Rappaport, editor of *Information for Decision Making: Quantitative and Behavioral Dimensions* (Prentice-Hall, 1975). The book contains Rappaport's chapter on discounted cash flow, the point of which is to maximize the immediate value of investment projects "subject to the constraint that the earnings of the company must grow at a stipulated rate." Also see Swinburn BA, et al. The global obesity pandemic: Shaped by global drivers and local environments. *Lancet* 2011;378:804–14.

14. Nestle M. *Food Politics: How the Food Industry Influences Nutrition and Health*, revised edition. Berkeley: U California Press, 2007. Nestle M, et al. Behavioral and social influences on food choice. *Nutrition Reviews* 1998;56(5):s50–s74.

15. Rosenheck R. Fast food consumption and increased caloric intake: A systematic review of a trajectory towards weight gain and obesity risk. *Obesity Reviews* 2008;9:535–37. Potti JM, Popkin BM. Trends in energy intake among US children by eating location and food source. *JADA* 2011;111:1156–64. Todd JE, Mancino L, Lin B-H. The impact of food away from home on diet quality. USDA Economic Research Report No. 90, February 2010.

16. USDA. Food marketing system in the U.S.: New product introductions, May 21, 2010, at www.ers.usda.gov/Briefing/FoodMarketingSystem/new_product.htm. Reedy J, Krebs-Smith SM. Dietary sources of energy, solid fats, and added sugars among children and adolescents in the United States. *JADA* 2010;110:1477–84.

17. Young LR, Nestle M. The contribution of increasing portion sizes to the obesity epidemic. *Am J Public Health* 2002;92:246–49. Young LR, Nestle M. Portion sizes and obesity: Responses of the fast-food companies. *J Public Health Policy*

2007;28:238–48. Rolls BJ, Morris EL, Roe LS. Portion size of food affects energy intake in normal-weight and overweight men and women. *AJCN* 2002;76:1207–13. Wansink B, van Ittersum K. Portion size me: Downsizing our consumption norms. *JADA* 2007;107:1103–6. Diliberti N, et al. Increased portion size leads to increased energy intake in a restaurant meal. *Obesity Res* 2004;12:562–68.

18. Farley TA, et al. The ubiquity of energy-dense snack foods: A national multi-city study. *Am J Public Health* 2010;100:306–11.

19. Piernas C, Popkin BM. Trends in snacking among U.S. children. *Health Affairs* 2010;29(3):398–404. Duffey KJ, Popkin BM. Energy density, portion size, and eating occasions: Contributions to increased energy intake in the United States, 1977–2006. *PLoS Medicine* 8(6):e1001050, June 28, 2011.

20. Davis B, Carpenter C. Proximity of fast-food restaurants to schools and adolescent obesity. *Am J Public Health* 2009;99:505–10. Painter JE, Wansink B, Hieggelke JB. How visibility and convenience influence candy consumption. *Appetite* 2002;38(3):237–38. Anonymous. Dispensing junk: How school vending undermines efforts to feed children well. CSPI, May 2004, online at www.cspinet.org/new/pdf/dispensing_junk.pdf.

21. Monsivais P, Aggarwal A, Drewnowski A. Following federal guidelines to increase nutrient consumption may lead to higher food costs for consumers. *Health Affairs* 2011;30(8):1–7. Leonhardt D. Sodas a tempting tax target. *NYT*, May 19, 2009, at www.nytimes.com/2009/05/20/business/economy/20leonhardt.html, and What's wrong with this chart? *NYT*, May 20, 2009, at http://economix.blogs.ny times.com/2009/05/20/whats-wrong-with-this-chart. But see Kuchler F, Stewart H. Price trends are similar for fruit, vegetables, and snack foods. USDA, Economic Research Service, Economic Research Report No. 55, March 2008, available at www .ers.usda.gov/publications/err55/err55.pdf. These USDA economists argue that Consumer Price Index data overstate the rise in the indexed price of fruits and vegetables. Andreyeva T, Brownell KD. The impact of food prices on consumption: A systematic review of research on the price elasticity of demand for food. *Am J Public Health* 2010;100:216–22.

22. 100 leading national advertisers, 2010. *Advertising Age*, June 20, 2010. Wansink B, Chandon P. Can "low-fat" nutrition labels lead to obesity? *J Marketing Res* 2006;43:605–17. Wansink B. *Mindless Eating: Why We Eat More than We Think*. New York: Bantam, 2006:1.

23. Kessler DA. *The End of Overeating*. Emmaus, PA: Rodale, 2009.

22. MORE CALORIE CONFUSION: PORTION DISTORTION, HEALTH HALOS, AND WISHFUL THINKING

1. Burros M. Losing count of calories as plates fill up. *NYT*, April 2, 1997.

2. Backstrand J, et al. *Fat Chance*. Washington, DC: Center for Science in the Public Interest, 1997.

3. Wansink B, Cheney MM. Super bowls: Serving bowl size and food consumption. *JAMA* 2005;293(14):1727–28.

4. Carels RA, Konrad K, Harper J. Individual differences in food perceptions and calorie estimation: An examination of dieting status, weight, and gender. *Appetite* 2007;49:450–58.

5. Chandon P, Wansink B. The biasing health halos of fast-food restaurant health claims: Lower calorie estimates and higher side-dish consumption intentions. *J Consumer Res* 2007;34:301–14.

6. Aydinoğlu NZ, Krishna A. Guiltless gluttony: The asymmetric effect of size labels on size perceptions and consumption. *J Consumer Res* 2011;37:1095–112.

7. Schuldt J, Schwarz N. The "organic" path to obesity? Organic claims influence calorie judgments and exercise recommendations. *Judgment and Decision Making* 2010;5:144–50.

8. Lavienja AJLM, et al. Determinants of obesity-related underreporting of energy intake. *Am J Epidemiology* 1998;147:1081–86. Wansink B, Chandon P. Meal size, not body size, explains errors in estimating the calorie content of meals. *Annals of Internal Medicine* 2006;145:326–32. Chandon P, Wansink B. Is obesity caused by calorie underestimation? A psychophysical model of meal size estimation. *J Marketing Res* 2007;44:84–99. Muhlheim L, et al. Do unsuccessful dieters intentionally underreport food intake? *Int'l J Eating Disorders* 1998;24:259–66.

9. Kellogg School of Management. The dieter's paradox. News release, September 20, 2010. Chernev A. The dieter's paradox. *J Consumer Psychology* 2011;21:178–83.

10. Retherford M. *The Negative Calorie Diet.* Self-published. Kindle edition, available at www.negativecaloriediet.com. No publication date is given other than a mention that the book first appeared in 1997. Also see: Vaughn CL. *Bulk Up Your Diet with Negative Calorie Foods.* Kindle edition, Alleywolf.com, 2011.

11. Rolls BJ. *The Volumetrics Eating Plan: Techniques and Recipes for Feeling Full on Fewer Calories.* New York: Harper, 2007. Upton J. Metabolism myths—busted. *Prevention* 2008;10(60):83–89.

12. International Food Information Council Foundation. *2011 Food and Health Survey,* May 5, 2011, available at www.foodinsight.org/Resources/Detail.aspx?topic =2011_Food_Health_Survey_Consumer_Attitudes_Toward_Food_Safety_ Nutrition_Health.

13. Hellmich N. Study: Americans mostly clueless when it comes to calories. *USA Today,* July 7, 2010.

23. CALORIE LABELING: SCIENCE AND POLITICS

1. Early Rice Krispies cereals listed ingredients as rice, malt, sugar, and salt. The sugar was sucrose. In 1982 Kellogg replaced some of the sugar with corn syrup. It replaced corn syrup with high fructose corn syrup (HFCS) in 1996. Negative perceptions of HFCS caused the company to revert to sucrose in 2010. Added vitamins

and minerals constituted the one other ingredient change but these are not sources of calories.

2. Park Y, et al. History of cereal-grain product fortification in the United States. *Nutrition Today* 2001;36:124–37. White House Conference on Food, Nutrition and Health. *Final Report.* Washington, DC: U.S. Government Printing Office, 1970, online at www.nns.nih.gov/1969/full_report/White_House_Report2_S1a.pdf.

3. Food labeling regulations: The official summary of the regulations published in the *Federal Register,* January 19, 1973. *Nutrition Today* 1973;8(1):14–15.

4. Kellogg Company. *A Citizen's Petition: The Relationship between Diet and Health.* Battle Creek, MI: Kellogg Co. Submitted May 22, 1985, to Dockets Management Branch, FDA. For a brief history of nutrition labeling policy, see: Wartella EA, Lichtenstein AH, Boon CS, eds. *Examination of Front-of-Package Nutrition Rating Systems and Symbols: Phase 1 Report.* Washington, DC: National Academies Press, 2010. Sullivan is quoted in: Hilts PJ. U.S. plans to make sweeping changes in labels on food. *NYT,* March 8, 1990.

5. FDA. Food labeling: Final rules. *FR* 1993;58:2066–941. For USDA-regulated foods, see chapter 25.

6. FDA, *FR* 1993;58:2082.

7. Code of Federal Regulations. Title 21: Food and Drugs, Part 101—Food Labeling, Section 101.9, Nutrition labeling of food, available at www.accessdata.fda.gov/scripts/cdrh/cfdocs/cfCFR/CFRSearch.cfm?fr=101.9.

8. FDA, *FR* 1993;58:2111.

9. FDA, *FR* 1993;58:2246.

10. HHS. *The Surgeon General's Report on Nutrition and Health.* Washington, DC: U.S. Government Printing Office, 1988. IOM. *Diet and Health.* Washington, DC: National Academies Press, 1989.

11. Marion Nestle discusses this history and the SnackWell phenomenon in her books *Food Politics* (rev. ed. 2007) and *What to Eat* (2007).

12. FDA, *FR* 1993;58:2217–18.

13. The figure was a population-weighted average for people age four and over, based on the most recent census data of that time. Christine Taylor, personal communication, September 12, 2010. Dr. Taylor was the FDA official of record on the 1993 *FR* documents.

14. FDA. How to understand and use the Nutrition Facts label, revised November 2004, at www.fda.gov/Food/LabelingNutrition/ConsumerInformation/ucm078889.htm#see2.

15. For health claims, see: FDA. Claims that can be made for conventional foods and dietary supplements, September 2003, at www.fda.gov/food/labelingnutrition/labelclaims/ucm111447.htm. For nutrient content claims, see: FDA. *Food Labeling Guide.* Appendix A: Definitions of nutrient content claims, guidance for industry: A food labeling guide, October 2009, at www.fda.gov/Food/GuidanceCompliance RegulatoryInformation/GuidanceDocuments/FoodLabelingNutrition/Food LabelingGuide/ucm064911.htm.

24. ALCOHOL LABELS: INDUSTRY VS. CONSUMERS

1. The history of the TTB is complicated. From its inception, the Bureau of Alcohol, Tobacco and Firearms (ATF) was part of the Treasury Department. It remained there until 2002, when the Homeland Security Act divided it into two parts: the Bureau of Alcohol, Tobacco, Firearms and Explosives (still called the ATF) and the Alcohol and Tobacco Tax and Trade Bureau (TTB). In January 2003 the ATF was moved out of Treasury and into the Justice Department to better cope with enforcement issues related to the illegal alcohol trade. The TTB remains in Treasury, where it is responsible for the revenues and regulation of legal alcoholic beverages.

2. CSPI's alcohol policy home page is at www.cspinet.org/alcohol/index.html. Its alcohol ingredient and nutrition labeling home page is at www.cspinet.org/booze/iss_ingred_label.htm. The CSPI documents discussed in this chapter were accessible through that site in 2011.

3. See: TTB. Labeling: Laws and regulations, at www.ttb.gov/labeling/laws_and_regs.shtml. Barley is a grain. Hops derive from a flower used for flavoring. FDA. Guidance for industry: Labeling of certain beers subject to the labeling jurisdiction of the Food and Drug Administration: Draft guidance, August 2009, available at www.fda.gov/Food/GuidanceComplianceRegulatoryInformation/Guidance Documents/FoodLabelingNutrition/ucm166239.htm. TTB. TTB ruling no. 2008-3: Classification of brewed products as "beer" under the Internal Revenue Code of 1986 and as "malt beverages" under the Federal Alcohol Administration Act, July 7, 2008. FR 2008;139:41259–61.

4. Code of Federal Regulations—Title 27. Alcohol, Tobacco Products and Firearms. 27 CFR 7.26—Alcohol content (suspended as of April 19, 1993; see §7.71) at TTB. Trade practices: Federal Alcohol Administration Act, at http://cfr.vlex.com/vid/alcoholic-content-suspended-april-see-71-19671301.

5. Adolph Coors Co. v. Nicholas Brady et al. U.S. Court of Appeals, Tenth Circuit. Sept. 23, 1991, at http://law.justia.com/cases/federal/appelate-courts/F2/944/1543/34860/.

6. Rubin v. Coors Brewing Co. (93-1631), 514 U.S. 476 (1995). ATF. Alcoholic content labeling for malt beverages. FR 1993;58:21228–33.

7. CSPI was founded in 1971. It soon published Michael F. Jacobson's *Eater's Digest: The Consumer's Factbook of Food Additives* (Garden City, NY: Doubleday, 1972).

8. ATF. Labeling and advertising of wine, distilled spirits and malt beverages. FR 1980;45:40538–53. The history of alcohol calorie and ingredient labeling since 1972 is recounted in: ATF. Advance notice of proposed rulemaking: Labeling and advertising of wines, distilled spirits and malt beverages; request for public comment. FR 2005;70:22274–83.

9. Nestle M. *Food Politics: How the Food Industry Influences Nutrition and Health*, revised edition. Berkeley: U California Press, 2007:84–91. The 2010 Dietary Guidelines say, "If alcohol is consumed, it should be consumed in moderation—up to one

drink per day for women and two drinks per day for men—and only by adults of legal drinking age." See: USDA, HHS. *Dietary Guidelines for Americans, 2010,* 7th ed. Washington, DC: U.S. Government Printing Office, December 2010:21, available at www.cnpp.usda.gov/DietaryGuidelines.htm.

10. FDA. Caffeinated alcoholic beverages, November 17, 2010, at www.fda.gov/Food/FoodIngredientsPackaging/ucm190366.htm.

11. MillerCoors lists percent alcohol, calories, carbohydrates, protein, sodium, and fats on its website at www.millercoors.com. Most of its products provide 100 to 150 calories per 12 ounces, but some Sparks products provide 250 or more.

12. ATF. Advance notice of proposed rulemaking: Nutrition labeling for wine, distilled spirits and malt beverages; request for public comment. *FR* 1993;58:42517–18.

13. Quoted in ATF, *FR* 2005;70:22278.

14. CSPI. Petition to improve mandatory label information on alcoholic beverages ("Alcohol Facts"), December 16, 2003:6–7.

15. TTB. Serving Facts information on alcohol beverages. Available at the CSPI Alcohol Policies Project, at www.cspinet.org/booze/TTBServingsFactsWhitePaper.pdf. See also: TTB, *FR*2005;70:22274–83.

16. Nigro D. Diageo to begin selling wines as "low-carb." *Wine Spectator,* April 20, 2004. Nestle quoted in: Day S. Diageo to put nutrition labels on liquor. *NYT,* December 18, 2003.

17. Hacker GA, Cohen B. Comments of Center for Science in the Public Interest to the Alcohol and Tobacco Tax and Trade Bureau on the labeling and advertising of wines, distilled spirits and malt beverages, September 23, 2005, available at www.cspinet.org/booze/2005/pdf/CSPI_Comments_on_TTB_IngLabeling.pdf.

18. TTB. Labeling and advertising of wines, distilled spirits and malt beverages; proposed rule. *FR* 2007;72:41860–84.

19. Hacker G. Notice No. 73. Labeling and advertising of wines, distilled spirits, and malt beverages. Comment from Center for Science in the Public Interest (Hacker, George), January 22, 2008, available at www.regulations.gov/#!documentDetail;D=TTB-2007-0062-0261.

20. Marin Institute. The new spirits "thin-dustry," May 4, 2011, at www.marininstitute.org/site/blog/38-blog-entries/628-the-new-spirits-qthindustryq.html. The Skinnygirl margarita information is at www.skinnygirlcocktails.com/about-skinnygirl-margarita.php. Applebee's beverage menu is at www.applebees.com/Menu_Drinks.aspx.

25. WILL CALORIE LABELS HELP FIGHT OBESITY?

1. FDA. *Calories Count: Report of the Working Group on Obesity,* March 12, 2004. FDA. Questions and answers—The FDA's Obesity Working Group report, June 2, 2006. Both are available at www.fda.gov/Food/LabelingNutrition/ReportsResearch/ucm081114.htm. Quote: *Calories Count, Executive Summary.*

2. This history is recounted in two FDA notices: Food labeling; prominence of

calories: Proposed rule. *FR* 2005;70:17008–10. Food labeling: Serving sizes of products that can reasonably be consumed at one eating occasion; updating of Reference Amounts Commonly Consumed; approaches for recommending smaller portion sizes. *FR* 2005;70:17010–14.

3. Coca-Cola. Press release: The Coca-Cola company announces worldwide commitment to place energy information on front of product packaging, September 30, 2009. Coca-Cola. Advertisement (full page). *NYT,* February 10, 2011:A11. The ad reads, "Calorie information at your fingertips. . . . We're working together to provide calorie information right up front, so you can choose what's right for you. www .ClearOnCalories.Org." It was signed by Coca-Cola, Dr. Pepper/Snapple, PepsiCo, SunnyD, and the American Beverage Association.

4. FDA. Agency information collection activities; proposed collection; comment request; experimental study of nutrition facts label formats. *FR* 2009;74:59553–54. FDA. Background information on point of purchase labeling, October 2009, at www.fda.gov/Food/LabelingNutrition/LabelClaims/ucm187320.htm. FDA. Agency information collection activities; submission for office of management and budget review; comment request; experimental studies of nutrition symbols on food packages. *FR* 2009;229:62786–92. FDA. New front-of-package labeling initiative, updated March 3, 2010, at www.fda.gov/Food/LabelingNutrition/ucm202726.htm.

5. FDA. Agency information collection activities: Proposed collection; comment request; internet survey on barriers to food label use. *FR* 2009;74:42676–77. Wartella EA, Lichtenstein AH, Boon CS, eds. *Examination of Front-of-Package Nutrition Rating Systems and Symbols: Phase 1 Report,* Washington, DC: National Academies Press, 2010. Wartella EA, et al., eds. *Front-of-Package Nutrition Rating Systems and Symbols: Promoting Healthier Choices.* Washington, DC: National Academies Press, 2011. FDA. Front-of-pack and shelf tag nutrition symbols; establishment of docket; request for comments and information. *FR* 2010;75:22602–6.

6. Lin C-T J, Levy A. Food and Drug Administration front-of-pack consumer research. Report presented at IOM, Food and Nutrition Board, October 26, 2010. This information is summarized in chapter 5 of the second IOM report on front-of-package labels.

7. USDA. Nutrition labeling of meat and poultry products. *FR* 1993;58:632–35.

8. USDA. Nutrition labeling of single-ingredient products and ground or chopped meat and poultry products: Final rule. *FR* 2010;75:82148–67.

9. Much of this part of the chapter comes from: Nestle M. Health care reform in action—calorie labeling goes national. *NEJM* 2010;362:2343–45. See also: Patient Protection and Affordable Care Act of 2010, Pub. L. No. 111-148 (March 23, 2010), Section 4205: Nutrition labeling of standard menu items at chain restaurants:455–58. Available at www.gpo.gov/fdsys/pkg/PLAW-111publ148/pdf/PLAW-111publ148 .pdf.

10. CSPI. Anyone's guess: The need for nutrition labeling at fast-food and other chain restaurants, November 2003, available at www.cspinet.org/restaurantreport .pdf.

11. FDA. Backgrounder: The Keystone Forum on away-from-home foods: Opportunities for preventing weight gain and obesity, June 2, 2006, available at www .fda.gov/Food/LabelingNutrition/ReportsResearch/ucm081114.htm.

12. Larson N, Story M. *Menu Labeling: Does Providing Nutrition Information at the Point of Purchase Affect Consumer Behavior?* Princeton, NJ: Robert Wood Johnson Foundation, June 2009.

13. Farley TA, et al. New York City's fight over calorie labeling. *Health Affairs* 2009;28:w1098–w1109.

14. Elbel B, et al. Calorie labeling and food choices: A first look at the effects on low-income people in New York City. *Health Affairs* 2009;28:w1110–w1121. Elbel B, Gyamfi J, Kersh R. Child and adolescent fast-food choice and the influence of calorie labeling: A natural experiment. *Int'l J Obesity* 2011;35:493–500. Morrison RM, Mancino L, Variyam JN. Will calorie labeling in restaurants make a difference? *Amber Waves*, March 2011, online at www.ers.usda.gov/AmberWaves/March11/Features/CalorieLabeling.htm.

15. Bernstein S. Restaurants revamping menus in response to calorie labeling rules. *Los Angeles Times*, June 22, 2011. Dumanovsky T, et al. Changes in energy content of lunchtime purchases from fast food restaurants after introduction of calorie labeling: Cross sectional customer surveys. *BMJ* 2011;343:d4464, online at www.bmj .com/content/343/bmj.d4464.

16. Urban LE, et al. Accuracy of stated energy contents of restaurant foods. *JAMA* 2011;306:287–93.

17. FDA. Disclosure of nutrient content information for standard menu items offered for sale at chain restaurants or similar retail food establishments and for articles of food sold from vending machines. *FR* 2010;75:39026–28. FDA documents on menu labeling are available on its web page "New Menu and Vending Machines Labeling Requirements," at www.fda.gov/Food/LabelingNutrition/ucm217762 .htm. The "Draft Guidance for Industry" was issued on August 24, 2010. The FDA withdrew it on January 21, 2011, and issued separate sets of proposed rules for restaurants and vending machines on April 6, 2011, available at www.fda.gov/food/labeling nutrition/default.htm.

18. Loewenstein G. Confronting reality: Pitfalls of calorie posting. *AJCN* 2011;93:679–80.

CONCLUSION: HOW TO COPE WITH THE CALORIE ENVIRONMENT

1. Van Wormer JJ, et al. Self weighing promotes weight loss for obese adults. *Am J Preventive Medicine* 2009;36:70–73. Hall KD, Chow CC. Estimating changes in free-living energy intake and its confidence interval. *AJCN* 2011;94:66–74.

2. Atwater WO. *Foods: Nutritive Value and Cost.* USDA Farmers' Bull No. 23, 1894:25.

3. Jacobson MF. *Liquid Candy: How Soft Drinks Are Harming Americans' Health.* Washington, DC: CSPI, 2005.

4. USDA, HHS. *Dietary Guidelines for Americans, 2010*, 7th ed. Washington, DC: U.S. Government Printing Office, December 2010:21, available at www.cnpp .usda.gov/DietaryGuidelines.htm.

5. USDA released its new food guide, MyPlate, June 2, 2011, at www.choosemy plate.gov. This guide replaces the 2005 MyPyramid.

6. Roberto CA, et al. Influence of licensed characters on children's taste and snack preferences. *Pediatrics* 2010;126:88–93.

7. CDC. Physical activity for everyone. How much physical activity do adults need? February 16, 2011, at www.cdc.gov/physicalactivity/everyone/guidelines/index .html.

8. Yancey T. *Instant Recess: Building a Fit Nation 10 Minutes at a Time*. Berkeley: U California Press, 2010.

9. Dietz WH, Gortmaker SL. Do we fatten our children at the television set? Obesity and television viewing in children and adolescents. *Pediatrics* 1985;75:807–12. Wiecha JL, et al. When children eat what they watch: Impact of television viewing on dietary intake in youth. *Archives of Pediatric and Adolescent Medicine* 2006;160:436–42. Mink M, et al. Nutritional imbalance endorsed by televised food advertisements. *JADA* 2010;110:904–10. Henry J. Kaiser Family Foundation. Generation M²: Media in the lives of 8- to 18-year-olds, January 2010, at www.kff.org/ entmedia/mho12010pkg.cfm. Foster JA, Gore SA, West DS. Altering TV viewing habits: An unexplored strategy for adult obesity intervention. *Am J Health Behavior* 2006;30:3–14. Hu FB, et al. Television watching and other sedentary behaviors in relation to risk of obesity and type 2 diabetes mellitus in women. *JAMA* 2003;289:1785–91.

10. Adapted from: Nestle M, Jacobson MF. Halting the obesity epidemic: A public health policy approach. *Public Health Reports* 2000;115:12–24.

11. Marion Nestle writes about such issues and provides links to organizations working on many areas of food and nutrition policy on her blog at www.foodpolitics. com and on Twitter @marionnestle. For recommendations for national and international government action, see Gortmaker SL, et al. Changing the future of obesity: Science, policy, and action. *Lancet* 2011;378:838–47.

APPENDIX ONE: SELECTED EVENTS IN THE HISTORY OF CALORIES, 1614–1919

1. Dates for older events are approximate. Principal sources: Carpenter KJ. A short history of nutritional science: Part 2. *J Nutrition* 2003;133:975–84. Hargrove JL. Does the history of food energy units suggest a solution to "Calorie confusion"? *Nutrition J* 2007;6(Dec 17):44, available at www.nutritionj.com/content/6/1/ 44. Lusk G. *Clio Medica X. Nutrition*. New York: Paul B. Hoeber, 1933. McCollum EV. *A History of Nutrition*. Boston: Houghton Mifflin, 1957:115–33. Todhunter EN. Chronology of some events in the development and application of the science of nutrition. *Nutrition Reviews* 1976;34(12):353–65.

APPENDIX TWO: THE RESPIRATORY QUOTIENT (RQ)

1. Livesey G, Elia M. Estimation of energy expenditure, net carbohydrate utilization, and net fat oxidation and synthesis by indirect calorimetry: Evaluation of errors with special reference to the detailed composition of fuels. *AJCN* 1988;47:608–28.

2. Jebb SA, et al. Changes in macronutrient balance during over- and underfeeding assessed by 12-d continuous whole-body calorimetry. *AJCN* 1996;64:259–66.

APPENDIX THREE: FREQUENTLY ASKED QUESTIONS

1. Wrangham R. *Catching Fire: How Cooking Made Us Human.* New York: Basic Books, 2010. Englyst HN, Cummings J. Digestion of the polysaccharides of some cereal foods in the human small intestine. *AJCN* 1985;42:778–87. Fleming SE, Vose JR. Digestibility of raw and cooked starches from legume seeds using the laboratory rat. *J Nutrition* 1979;109:2067–75. Leonard WR, Snodgrass JJ, Robertson ML. Effects of brain evolution on human nutrition and metabolism. *Annual Review of Nutrition* 2007;27:311–27.

2. Kokkinos A, et al. Eating slowly increases the postprandial response of the anorexigenic gut hormones, peptide YY and glucagon-like peptide-1. *J Clinical Endocrinology and Metabolism* 2010;95:333–37. Maruyama K, et al. The joint impact on being overweight of self-reported behaviors of eating quickly and eating until full: Cross sectional survey. *British Medical J* 2008;337:a2002, online at www.bmj.com/content/337/bmj.a2002.full. Andrade AM, Greene GW, Melanson KJ. Eating slowly led to decreases in energy intake within meals in healthy women. *JADA* 2008;108:1186–91. Lemmens SG, et al. Staggered meal consumption facilitates appetite control without affecting postprandial energy intake. *J Nutrition* 2011;141:482–88.

3. Stiles PG. Horace Fletcher (obituary). *Am J Public Health* 1919;9(3):210–11, available at www.ncbi.nlm.nih.gov/pmc/articles/PMC1362489/pdf/amjphealth00211-0050.pdf. Li J, et al. Improvement in chewing activity reduces energy intake in one meal and modulates plasma gut hormone concentrations in obese and lean young Chinese men. *AJCN* 2011;94:709–16.

4. Wyatt HR, et al. Long-term weight loss and breakfast in subjects in the National Weight Control Registry. *Obesity Research* 2002;10:78–82. De Castro, JM. The time of day of food intake influences overall intake in humans. *J Nutrition* 2004;134:104–11. Levitsky DA. The non-regulation of food intake in humans: Hope for reversing the epidemic of obesity. *Physiology and Behavior* 2005;86:623–32. Schusdziarra V, et al. Impact of breakfast on daily energy intake—an analysis of absolute versus relative breakfast calories. *Nutrition J* 2011;10:5, available at www.nutritionj.com/content/10/1/5.

5. Kellogg. Special K Challenge, at www.specialk.com/challenge/reso.

6. Rolls BJ, et al. Time course of effects of preloads high in fat or carbohydrate on food intake and hunger ratings in humans. *Am J Physiology* 1991;260:R756–63.

Chapelot, D. The role of snacking in energy balance: A biobehavioral approach. *J Nutrition* 2011;141:158–62.

7. Rolls BJ, et al. Energy density but not fat content of foods affected energy intake in lean and obese women. *AJCN* 1999;69:863–71. Prentice AM, Jebb SA. Fast foods, energy density, and obesity: A possible mechanistic link. *Obesity Reviews* 2003;4:187–94. Kessler DA. *The End of Overeating.* Emmaus, PA: Rodale, 2009. American Institute for Cancer Research. Experts fact-check "McDonald's diet" story, June 23, 2008, at www.aicr.org/site/News2?page=NewsArticle&id=13201 &news_iv_ctrl=0&abbr=pr_.

8. Forbes GB. Do obese individuals gain weight more easily than non-obese individuals? *AJCN* 1990;52:224–27.

9. Ioannides-Demos LL, Piccenna L, McNeil JJ. Pharmacotherapies for obesity: Past, current and future therapies. *J Obesity* 2011;2011:179674. Epub December 12, 2010, at www.ncbi.nlm.nih.gov/pubmed/21197148. Weight-control Information Network (WIN). Prescription medicines for the treatment of obesity, updated December 2010, at http://win.niddk.nih.gov/publications/prescription.htm.

10. Ballinger A. Orlistat in the treatment of obesity. *Expert Opinion on Pharmacotherapy* 2000;1:841–47.

11. MedlinePlus. Orlistat, at www.nlm.nih.gov/medlineplus/druginfo/meds/a601244.html. Torgerson JJ, et al. Xenical in the Prevention of Diabetes in Obese Subjects (XENIDOS) Study. *Diabetes Care* 2004;27:155–61.

12. Livingston EH. The incidence of bariatric surgery has plateaued in the U.S. *Am J Surgery* 2010;200:378–85. Roux CW, et al. Gut hormones as mediators of appetite and weight loss after Roux-en-Y gastric bypass. *Annals of Surgery* 2007;246:780–85. Robinson MK. Surgical treatment of obesity—weighing the facts. *NEJM* 2009;361:520–21. Maggard MA, et al. Meta-analysis: Surgical treatment of obesity. *Annals of Internal Medicine* 2005;142:547–59. Pinkney JH, Johnson AB, Gale AM. The big fat bariatric bandwagon. *Diabetologia* 2010;53:1815–22. For a comment on bariatric surgery in young people see Inglefinger JR. Bariatric surgery in adolescents. *NEJM* 2011;365:1365–67.

13. See, for example, Diabetes Monitor—Calories don't count, January 6, 2010, at www.diabetesmonitor.com/calories.htm.

LIST OF TABLES

271

LIST OF FIGURES

ACKNOWLEDGMENTS

As with all such projects, we could not have done this without assistance from colleagues, friends, and family. Our first thanks go to Stan Holwitz, Marion Nestle's long-time editor at University of California Press, for suggesting that we try to address public confusion about calories and their effects.

For providing critical information, documents, and explanations not readily available elsewhere, we thank Roger Bagnell, André Bensadoun, Celeste Clark, Ellen Fried, George Hacker, Corinna Hawkes, Rashid Kerdouch, Robert Lange, Michele Simon, Lisa Sutherland, Christine Taylor, Fred Tripp, Brian Wansink, and Lisa Young. We particularly thank Arthur Resnick for clarifying the intricacies of alcohol regulation two days before he retired from the Alcohol and Tobacco Tax and Trade Bureau.

Our NYU and Cornell colleagues Beth Dixon, David Levitsky, and Per Pinstrup-Anderson read and commented on some of the knottier sections of the book. We have nothing but admiration for other colleagues—Joanne Csete, Maya Joseph, and David Ludwig—who read our initial manuscript in its entirety, and for Carolyn Dimitri, Rebecca Nestle, Domingo Piñero, and Lisa Sasson, who read through the page proofs with eagle eyes. We hope it is evident that we listened carefully and acted on most of their thoughtful suggestions.

We thank Suzanne Natz and Domingo Piñero for technical support with some of the figures and are everlastingly grateful to Sheldon Watts for keeping Marion Nestle's electronic life in good working order.

We are indebted to Daniel Fromson of Atlantic Life for his tutorial on how to write chapter titles. Everyone should have so inspiring a teacher. And it was a great pleasure—as always—to work with the talented and professional editorial, design, and production teams at UC Press.

Overall, we thank our administrators, colleagues, and students at New York University and Cornell University for their support of our work, and for granting Marion Nestle sabbatical leave to work on this book.

INDEX

Illustrations are indicated by *fig.* following the page reference. Tables are indicated by *t.* following the page reference.

CALIFORNIA STUDIES IN FOOD AND CULTURE

Darra Goldstein, Editor

TEXT
Jenson Pro 10.5/14

DISPLAY
Benton Gothic Regular and Light

COMPOSITOR
BookMatters, Berkeley

INDEXER
Kevin Millham

PRINTER AND BINDER
Maple-Vail Book Manufacturing Group